THE IMPLEMENTATION OF HEALTH PROMOTING SCHOOLS

Exploring the theories of what, why and how

Edited by
Oddrun Samdal and Louise Rowling

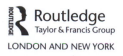

Routledge
Taylor & Francis Group

LONDON AND NEW YORK

First published 2013
by Routledge
2 Park Square, Milton Park, Abingdon, Oxon OX14 4RN

Simultaneously published in the USA and Canada
by Routledge
711 Third Avenue, New York, NY 10017

Routledge is an imprint of the Taylor & Francis Group, an informa business

British Library Cataloguing in Publication Data
A catalogue record for this book is available from the British Library

Library of Congress Cataloging in Publication Data
The implementation of health promoting schools : exploring the theories of what, why and how / [edited by] Oddrun Samdal, Louise Rowling.
 p. cm.
Includes index.
1. School hygiene—Cross-cultural studies. 2. Health education—Cross-cultural studies.
3. Health promotion—Cross-cultural studies. 4. School children—Health and hygiene.
5. School environment—Cross-cultural studies.
I. Samdal, Oddrun. II. Rowling, Louise.
LB3405.I482013
371.7′1—dc23
 2012024458

ISBN: 978–0–415–52554–1 (hbk)
ISBN: 978–0–415–52558–9 (pbk)
ISBN: 978–0–203–11979–2 (ebk)

Typeset in Bembo
by RefineCatch Limited, Bungay, Suffolk

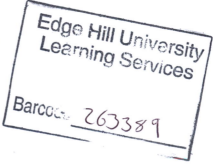

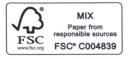

Printed and bound by CPI Group (UK) Ltd, Croydon, CR0 4YY

CONTENTS

PART II
Case studies   99

FIGURES AND TABLES

Figures

Tables

CONTRIBUTORS

Isabel Baptista, MED, is a Philologist with post-graduation training in Learning and Training Systems Management and is currently a researcher at the Technical University of Lisbon. She is the National Coordinator of the Health Education's Department in the Ministry of Education and Science (MEC). Isabel is also the representative of the MEC in several international organisations, for example Schools for Health in Europe (SHE) and the Gender Equality in Education Commission, and a member of the ministerial working group on Health and Sexual Education (2005–2007). Email: isabelbaptista@netcabo.pt

Margaret M. Barry is Professor of Health Promotion and Public Health and Head of the World Health Organization Collaborating Centre for Health Promotion Research at the National University of Ireland Galway. She has published widely in the field of mental health promotion and has worked closely with policymakers and practitioners on the development, implementation and evaluation of mental health promotion interventions and policies at national and international level. Margaret was elected as Global Vice President for Capacity Building, Education and Training by the International Union for Health Promotion and Education (2007–2010). She has acted as expert adviser on mental health promotion policy development in Canada, England, Ireland, Northern Ireland, New Zealand and Scotland. Email: margaret.barry@nuigalway.ie

Kevin Dadaczynski is a Research Fellow at the Center of Applied Health Science at the Leuphana University of Lüneburg. He has a diploma degree in health promotion and a master's degree in health psychology/health education. His research interests are: mental health of pupils, teachers and principals, health education and health promotion in schools and quality development and assurance in (school) health promotion and prevention. He is involved in

several national and international research projects. Email: dadaczynski@uni.
leuphana.de

Mark Dooris is Director of the Healthy Settings Unit and Reader in Health
and Sustainable Development within the School of Health at the University of
Central Lancashire (UCLan). Mark has a background in health promotion,
public health, community development, healthy cities and environmental and
transport policy – and has worked in a range of roles within the health service,
voluntary sector and local government. He has extensive experience in conducting
and managing action-focused research and carrying out health-related evaluations. Mark chaired the International Union of Health Promotion and Education's
Global Working Group on Healthy Settings from 2007–2012. Email: mtdooris@
uclan.ac.uk

Wolfgang Dür has a background in sociology, philosophy and law at the
University of Vienna. He is the Director of the Ludwig Boltzmann Institute for
Health Promotion Research in Vienna. His areas of work are medical curricula,
AIDS and sexual relations, systems analyses in health care, health promotion
research, evaluation, epidemiological research (children, adolescent, school), and
systems theory. He holds positions as Vice Chairman of the Austrian Society
for Public Health, Secretary of the Austrian Society for the Sociology of Health
and Medicine and is a Member of the Coordinating Committee of the
WHO-collaborative study 'Health Behaviour in School-aged Children' (HBSC;
www.hbsc.org). Email: wolfgang.duer@lbihpr.lbg.ac.at

Margarida Gaspar de Matos, PhD, is a Health and Clinical Psychologist,
Chartered Psychotherapist and Professor at the Department of Education at
the Technical University of Lisbon. She is also Coordinator of the Health
Education Research Unit and National Coordinator of International Research
Projects in the area of young people health promotion and national principal
investigator for several international research projects, among them 'Health
Behaviour in School-aged Children' (HBSC). Margarida was a member
of the ministerial working group of Health and Sexual Education
(2005–2007) and has broad experience in collaboration with Africa and
Latin America in the area of health promotion. Email: margaridagaspar@
netcabo.pt

Lisa Gugglberger is a Senior Researcher at the Ludwig Boltzmann Institute of
Health Promotion Research in Vienna, where for the past four years she has been
working in the field of health promoting schools. She is currently on secondment
at the University of Brighton, Centre for Health Research. In 2010 she spent four
months as a Visiting Researcher at the University of Edinburgh to carry out a
study about health promotion implementation in the Scottish school system. Lisa
is a trained sociologist, focused on qualitative research and evaluation. Her

research interests are health promotion implementation and capacity building for health promoting schools. Email: lisa.gugglberger@lbihpr.lbg.ac.at

Jo Inchley is Assistant Director of the Child and Adolescent Health Research Unit at the University of St Andrews, Scotland. Jo has worked in public health research for over 15 years and specialises in child and adolescent health and school health promotion. She was previously Evaluation Coordinator for the European Network of Health Promoting Schools in Scotland and is currently a member of the Schools for Health in Europe (SHE) research network. Jo has considerable experience of evaluating school-based interventions, particularly in the areas of nutrition and physical activity. Email: jci2@st-andrews.ac.uk

Evie Ledger is the current President of the Australian Health Promoting Schools Association. Her contribution to both the education and health sectors over 20 years includes leadership of many health promoting/whole school partnership initiatives in South Australia. Evie's work demonstrates her significant commitment to numerous health promoting school partnership activities through the development and delivery of state wide strategies, professional learning, and development of support materials for health, education, care, sport, recreation and community sectors as well as co-authoring a number of published educational resources. Evie has presented at international, national and state conferences both in Australia and overseas to a variety of audiences and received international awards for innovative projects. Email: evieledger@yahoo.com

Colin Noble, initially a teacher of history and physical education, began one of the first healthy school programmes in the UK in 1990 when working for Kirklees Local Education Authority in Yorkshire. Since then he has written a number of articles about healthy schools. He joined the National Healthy Schools Programme team in 2001, was the National Coordinator from 2004 to 2007 and oversaw a major revision to the Programme in 2005. The author of books about boys' achievement, personal social and health education and pupil responsibility, Colin is now an educational consultant. Email: colinnoble@ntlworld.com

Peter Paulus works as a Professor at the Institute of Psychology at the Leuphana University of Lüneburg. His work focuses on the following areas: educational psychology, family psychology, health psychology, education, counselling, and health promotion. He heads the research of several nationwide projects relating to school health promotion: 'MindMatters – mit psychischer Gesundheit gute Schule machen' (MindMatters – Promotion of mental health in secondary schools) (2002–2012), 'Lernen mit Gefühl. Mit psychischer Gesundheit gute Schule machen – Primarbereich' (Learning with emotion. Promotion of good school through mental health – primary schools) (2007–2012),

'Kompetenzzentrum: Psychische Gesundheit in Bildung und Erziehung' (Competence Center: Mental health in education) (2008–2013) and 'Ganztagsschulentwicklung und psychische Gesundheit' (Whole day school and mental health) (2010-2012). Email: paulus@uni.leuphana.de

Louise Rowling has been a teacher, school psychologist, academic and consultant. She is an honorary Associate Professor at the University of Sydney and has established over a 30-year period a national and international reputation for work on health promotion, particularly school health. Her areas of expertise include drug and alcohol education, health promoting schools, mental health and well-being and loss and grief. Louise was President of Australian Health Promoting Schools Association in its first formative five years and in that role was Director of the National Health Promoting Schools Initiative in 1997. She was the inaugural President of 'Intercamhs', the International Alliance of Child and Adolescent Mental Health and Schools, for five years. She was co-director of the research and development phase of MindMatters, the national mental health promotion project that uses the health promoting school as an underlying framework. Email: louise.rowling@sydney.edu.au

Oddrun Samdal is a Professor at the Department of Health Promotion and Development at the University of Bergen. She is an educator by training and has for 20 years conducted research, taught graduate courses and evaluated school-based interventions in the area of children and adolescents' life satisfaction, health and health-related behaviours. Oddrun was the Norwegian National Coordinator of the European Network of Health Promoting Schools from 1993 until 2009. Through this period she worked closely with national education and health authorities and schools to develop sustainable health promoting school practices. She is also the Databank Manager of the European and North American study 'Health Behaviour in School-aged Children. A WHO Cross-national survey'. Email: oddrun.samdal@uib.no

Daniel Sampaio, MD, PhD, is a Professor of psychiatry at the University of Lisbon Medical School. He is also a Senior Psychiatrist in the Department of Psychiatry at Santa Maria University Hospital in Lisbon. Daniel is a founder of the Portuguese Society for Family Therapy and has extensive research experience. He was the coordinator of the ministerial working group of Health and Sexual Education (2005–2007). Email: d.sampaio@netcabo.pt

Venka Simovska is a Professor and Research Director of the Programme for Health and Environmental Education at the Department of Education at Aarhus University, campus Copenhagen. Venka is a member of the International Planning Committee for the Schools for Health (SHE) network in Europe, and coordinator of the SHE Research Group related to the network. Her research is embedded within critical health education and health promotion in schools, focusing on student participation, empowerment and action competence, as well as teaching/learning processes related to health. Email: vs@dpu.dk

Hege Eikeland Tjomsland, PhD, is an Associate Professor at the Department of Education at the University of Bergen. She has long term experience in evaluating school-based intervention programmes aiming at promoting children's health, well-being and health–related behaviors. Her PhD and master's degrees were earned in health promotion with a particular focus on teachers' participation in health promoting schools. Today, her main research interests concern health promoting schools and young people's participation in physical activity both in physical education in school and in voluntary sports organisations. Email: hege.tjomsland@uib.no

Marilyn Toft is an experienced secondary school teacher and has worked extensively in a range of inner city schools. Leading a local authority's professional development programme, which included developing a successful local healthy schools network based on national and international experience, Marilyn instigated and, subsequently, directed the National Healthy Schools Programme in England, which was launched in 1999. Its success resulted in every local area achieving an accredited education and health partnership providing services to local schools. The principles of the programme remain embedded in school practice. Marilyn now provides consultancy services to schools and academies on improving behaviour and attendance, in the context of promoting well-being for all children and young people. Email: toftmarilyn@gmail.com

Nina Grieg Viig is an Associate Professor in pedagogics, and currently Dean of Research at Bergen University College, Faculty of Education, Norway. She has a MPhil and a PhD in Health Promotion, and her PhD thesis was part of the evaluation of the Norwegian Network of Health Promoting Schools. Her main research interests are within school health promotion and school development. Nina is involved in the European Network Schools for Health in Europe (SHE Network). She is a member of the Network's planning committee and research group. Email: Nina.Grieg.Viig@hib.no

Gloria Wells has provided organisational leadership in the Education, Human Services and Health sectors, with a specialised interest and responsibility for Health Promotion and Prevention for children and youth in communities and school-based settings in Alberta, Canada. She has 25 years successful experience in developing cross-sectoral collaboration processes and models at district and systems levels to operationalise a continuum of health and mental health programmes. This work has been under the umbrella of a Health Promoting Schools Framework, aimed at optimising learning outcomes by proactively addressing non-academic barriers to learning. She lives in British Columbia, Canada, and is currently the Executive Director of Wellsprings Education and

Human Service Consulting, and the President of the International Alliance for Child and Adolescent Mental Health in Schools Society (www.intercamhs.net). Email: wellsgl59@gmail.com

Bente Wold is a Professor at the Department of Health Promotion and Development at the University of Bergen, Norway. She is a trained psychologist, and completed her PhD in 1989. Her main research interests concern health promotion with young people, with a particular interest in positive youth development and health behaviours based on developmental, social and health psychology, as well as behavioural epidemiology. She has many years of experience in evaluation of school-based interventions, both with regard to health promoting schools and health promotion in schools. Email: bente.wold@uib.no

Barbara Woynarowska, M.D., Ph.D. is a Professor and Head of the Department of Biomedical and Psychological Basis of Education, Faculty of Pedagogy, Warsaw University. She is a member of the Committee of Human Development and Committee of Public Health, Polish Academy of Science. Former Principal Investigator in HBSC study (1990–2004) and national coordinator in European Network of Health Promoting Schools (1992–1997). She has 20 years' experience in the development of health promoting schools in Poland. She heads the Committee on Health Promotion and Prevention of Problems of Children and Adolescents (created by the Minister of National Education, Minister of Health, Minister of Sport and Tourism) and Head of the Chapter of the Health Promoting School National Certificate. Email: barwoy@pedagog.uw.edu.pl

Ian Young was Head of International Development at NHS Health Scotland, and is currently a school consultant for The International Union for Health Promotion and Education (IUHPE). Ian has 43 years of experience in Scotland as a high school teacher, educational adviser and health promoter in the NHS. He has extensive experience working with the World Health Organization, The Council of Europe, The European Commission, IUHPE, and Non-Governmental Organisations as a practitioner, researcher and writer. He has been involved in the health promoting schools movement in Europe since its inception in the early 1980s and has published over 30 peer-reviewed papers on the subject. He was awarded the honour of Member of the British Empire (MBE) in 2008 in Queen Elizabeth's Birthday Honours List in recognition of his work in school health promotion. Email: imyoung@blueyonder.co.uk

FOREWORD

The concept of the health promoting school emerged in the mid-1980s and was both a product of, and influence on, the evolution of health promotion as a distinct public health strategy. It has provided a framework for critical examination of actions to improve the health of school students and the wider school community, and has inspired a whole generation of creative thinking and experimentation over the past 25 years. Disappointingly, and despite this innovation, energy and enthusiasm, achieving successful implementation and sustaining the positive benefits for school students of school health programmes has proven to be challenging. After more than two decades, the implementation of the health promoting schools concept still lags some way behind the vision.

There are many reasons why this is the case – insufficient use has been made of promising theories that can provide structure and direction to the development of programmes; there is currently inadequate empirical research that can provide clear, evidence-based guidance on implementation; and there are significant philosophical and practical differences as to what is to be implemented and how, and what are the most appropriate measures of success in relation to a health promoting school. Although there are many excellent statements of principle, there is insufficient guidance on implementation in 'real life' conditions of schools.

This book fills key gaps in our understanding of the complex processes involved in introducing and sustaining an innovation in schools. It draws out the theoretical basis for health promotion in a school setting, makes good use of the emerging evidence from research, and uses case studies to provide practical guidance on implementation.

To achieve these outcomes the editors and authors recognise that schools are complex, evolving organisations that have to deal with many conflicting demands for time, resources and attention. The authors also explicitly recognise the practical difficulties of introducing and sustaining innovations such as health promoting schools into such a complex system.

The book draws extensively on experiences from a range of countries, and in doing so emphasises the importance of local context in the implementation of innovations. What emerges from this analysis is the need to be adaptable in implementation – understanding school culture; recognising that schools are first and foremost educational institutions; and acknowledging resource constraints and teacher capability as key factors influencing success and sustainability.

The case studies emphasise the significance of personal leadership, supporting policies, structures and networks. These examples also illustrate the importance of mutual respect and understanding between health and education agencies, and the need to mobilise the resources necessary to develop and sustain capacity for implementation within school systems.

The editors and authors bring unparalleled expertise and professional experience. There is a real sense that collectively they have 'lived' the experiences they describe, but have found a way to bring form and structure to these sometimes chaotic and unpredictable experiences.

The book also credibly identifies outstanding challenges, particularly the need for more and better research that examines both the process of introducing change, and how the impact and long term benefits of health promoting schools can be sustained.

In such a complex and context specific environment, it is hard to imagine an approach to the implementation of health promoting schools that will work in all circumstances. Progress in our understanding and practical experience tends to be more incremental. This book provides an excellent overview of important and relevant theory, research and practical experience that will allow the reader to select ideas with potential for application in a wide variety of different school contexts. In this way it provides a further important incremental step in translating the vision of a health promoting school into a practical reality.

Professor Don Nutbeam
University of Southampton

PREFACE

This book had its origin, as befitting a Norwegian–Australian collaboration, on Bondi beach, Sydney, Australia. We were having a conversation about our respective experiences of work in health promoting schools, in Norway and the European network of health promoting schools; and Australia and the World Health Organization, Western Pacific region. At that stage we calculated we had about 35 years of work experience on health promoting schools, between us. This book is the result of those years of experience, research and writing. We agreed that the 'black box', the area in most need of development, was implementation. There were guidelines and indicators but not a theoretically and empirically-based articulation of implementation.

Initially we planned to write an article. After three years of work this became two articles, but many times we both commented that we had enough material to write a book. The interest generated by presentations and then the publication of the articles about the eight components of implementation, prompted us to embark on this text. In writing and working with our contributors, our ideas have been conceptually refined. Health promoting schools was an initiative of the World Health Organization, so it is appropriate that we have drawn in other contributors for chapters and case studies from different parts of the world. This provides depth and richness.

Over the years, at national and international meetings, we met many devoted and excellent researchers and practitioners within health promoting schools. It has been a great asset for our work with the book to draw on their experiences and to be able to invite some of them to contribute as chapter and case study authors. Further, our close collaboration with schools, principals, teachers, students and school health services has both inspired and helped us in addressing not only what needs to be done when wanting to implement health promoting schools but also the importance of specifying why and how. We are thankful for what our work in the practice field taught us to look for and to develop in our research on implementation of health promoting schools. Our hope is that readers can benefit from this journey.

Oddrun Samdal and Louise Rowling

PART I

Theory base for implementation of health promoting schools

The first five chapters of this book articulate the development and main aims of health promoting schools as well as a theory base for implementation. Chapters 2 and 3 provide a more generic theoretical framework for settings based implementation demonstrating the need to address the complex interaction between individuals and organisations for successful implementation. Chapters 4 and 5 present concrete theory-driven implementation components for health promoting schools aiming to support practitioners to implement them with fidelity without losing flexibility for local adaptation needs.

1

INTRODUCTION

Oddrun Samdal and Louise Rowling

Health promoting schools – current status and needs for development

Whilst the health promoting school approach started out as an initiative from the health sector, it is today an initiative willingly taken on and developed by the education sector. The experience of schools has been that the focus on health promotion also stimulates the development of a good learning climate, so there is consistency between health promotion aims and school aims (Rowling & Jeffreys, 2000; Samdal, Viig & Wold, 2010; Tjomsland, Iversen & Wold, 2009; Viig & Wold, 2005).

The emergence of health promoting schools is nevertheless integrally linked with the disciplinary growth of health promotion and shifting priorities in schools. The formal establishment of health promotion is frequently considered to have taken place in 1986 with the publication of the Ottawa Charter for Health Promotion, an outcome of the first World Health Organization (WHO) conference on health promotion (WHO, 1986). In this document health promotion is defined as 'the process of enabling people to increase control over, and to improve, their health' (WHO, 1986). From the very beginning WHO's Regional Office in Europe introduced a settings approach to stimulate the development of health promotion (Kickbusch, 2003). Schools were considered one key setting to address, and the establish-ment of networks (national and multinational) of health promoting schools was used as a strategy to nurture the implementation of health promoting schools. The network approach led to the initiation of the European Network of Health Promoting Schools (known today as Schools for Health in Europe, www. schoolsforhealth.eu) and the Australian Health Promoting Schools Association (AHPSA), both established in 1992. Networks for health promoting schools have also been)established through WHO in the Western Pacific and Latin America.

However, the international health promotion impetus did not lead to uniform implementation (Clift, Bruun-Jensen & Paulus, 2005). The national approaches taken within the networks have varied a great deal from direct work with individual schools by establishing national networks of health promoting schools (e.g. Poland and United Kingdom), to primarily utilising policy strategies to initiate actions in schools through integrating the concept of health promoting schools in relevant White Papers and the national school curriculum (e.g. Denmark, Finland and Norway). The differences in national approaches were highly influenced by the national curriculum context, i.e. to what extent health education and health promotion were already core foci in national curriculums (Kickbusch, 2003). In Australia and the Scandinavian countries health education and health promotion were already mandatory curriculum areas. In other countries (for example the Netherlands) health related issues in school were mainly dealt with by health professionals. The Dutch focus continued to stimulate the role of the health sector encouraging a stronger link between the health and the education sector in this work (Leurs, Bessems, Schaalma & de Vries, 2007; Leurs *et al.*, 2005). Given the national differences in implementation we will in this book, present several case studies illustrating different implementation action of health promoting schools due to different contexts but with underlying similarities. The book in general and the case studies in particular apply the settings approach to health promoting schools as identified by WHO (Kickbusch, 2003), with a strong emphasis on the integration in an educational context, frequently known as a whole school approach. In this settings approach there is 'a desire to act in various ways on policies, re-shape environments, build partnerships, bring about sustainable change through participation, and develop empowerment and ownership of change through the setting' (Whitelaw *et al.*, 2001: 340–341) (for more details on the settings approach see Chapter 2).

Health promotion and health promoting schools is still a young field very much driven by policy and practice development. So far, little evidence exists as to the effectiveness of the health promoting school approach (Lister-Sharp, Chapman, Stewart-Brown & Sowden, 1999; Stewart-Brown, 2006). Building this evidence is critical to the further development of the field and the priority of governments to support it. A major challenge related to lack of evidence is vague operationalisation of what is to be implemented and how it should be implemented. While general guidelines articulating the principles of health promoting schools have been provided (see www.schoolsforhealth.eu; ENHPS, 1997; International Union for Health Promotion and Education (IUHPE), 2008, 2009; Tang *et al.*, 2009), their understanding and operationalisation have mainly been left to the schools, i.e. the practitioners. The lack of specific implementation guidelines makes it difficult for the schools to identify concrete actions to achieve a whole school health promotion approach and results in a wide array of practices across schools and countries. This further increases the challenge of establishing evidence of the health promoting school approach, as it is not clear what can be measured, nor how to manage the variety of actions taken.

Despite these challenges, IUHPE has identified a set of guidelines to facilitate the development of health promotion at school level:

1. Developing a supportive government/local authority policy for health promoting schools;
2. Achieving administrative and senior management support;
3. Creating a small group actively engaged in leading and coordinating actions including teachers, non-teaching staff, students, parents and community members;
4. Conducting an audit of current health promoting actions according to the essential elements;
5. Establishing agreed goals and a strategy to achieve them;
6. Developing a health promoting school charter;
7. Ensuring appropriate staff and community partners undertake capacity building programmes and that they have opportunities to put their skills into practice;
8. Celebrating milestones;
9. Completing specific goals;
10. Allowing three to four years to complete specific goals.
                    (International Union for Health Promotion and Education, 2008)

The science base for why these 10 steps are important is, however, not clear. This book concentrates on filling the gap in existing knowledge and practice. This next step in the refinement of effective health promoting schools sets out to delineate a science base for implementation components and detail guidelines for the actual implementation of the components.

Need for implementation guidelines of health promoting schools

Gaps in previous action mean that there is a strong need and support for creating a science base for the health promoting school approach. An important part of this work would be to articulate implementation components to guide schools in their work, i.e. a 'science of delivery' (Catford, 2009). Components are needed that propose 'models that can be put into practice in natural contexts' (Deschesnes, Couturier, Laberge & Campeau, 2010). Systematic identification of empirically and theoretically based components of quality implementation may then ensure efficient implementation of health promoting schools. Scientific knowledge of implementation and organisational development contributes to a theory base for this work. Additionally, reports documenting health promoting school practices constitute an important empirical base from which generic components can be extracted. Systematic identification and provision of clearly operationalised implementation components will allow practitioners to understand the function of each component so they can execute them with fidelity (Dusenbury, Brannigan, Falco & Hansen, 2003).

The absence of effective comprehensive implementation guidance for health promoting schools continually compromises the efficacy outcomes of whole school change for health and learning. In order to identify what and how to best implement the health promoting school initiative, a summary of the existing core principles, aims and structures is needed.

The core principles of health promoting schools

The first guidelines for health promoting schools go back to 1985 when WHO commissioned their collaborating centre, the Scottish Health Education Group (SHEG), to organise a European symposium on health promoting schools. This symposium identified three main elements of schools important to health promotion (Young, 2005):

* time allocated to health-related issues in the formal curriculum through subjects including home economics, physical education, social education and health studies;
* the hidden curriculum of the school including staff–pupil relationships, school–community relationships, the school environment and the quality of services such as school meals;
* the health and caring services providing a health promotion role in the school through screening, prevention and child guidance.

More recently the essence of a health promoting school approach has been summarised by the International Union for Health Promotion and Health Education (2008) and includes focus on:

1. school health policies – a written document stating the aims the school is striving towards within their health promoting effort;
2. physical environment of the school – should be safe and health promoting;
3. the social environment of the school – should ensure a well-functioning and inclusive psychosocial climate for students and staff;
4. the development of individual health skills and action competencies – emphasis should be placed on students developing essential life skills to help them take care of their own as well as others' physical, social and mental health;
5. school–community links – should ensure close collaboration between the school and the local community to make the best of the competence and resources available;
6. health services – should be a crucial partner in the development of a health promoting school.

Over the years, these principles have constituted the basis for the work in ongoing networks (St Leger, 2000), and represented at their initiation an important step beyond the previous curriculum focus on health education as the only means to influence and promote students' health. The presented foci are also in line with principles for comprehensive health in school outlined by the US Centers for Disease Control and Prevention (CDC) (see www.cdc.gov/HealthyYouth/CSHP/):

1. Health Education – a planned, sequential curriculum that addresses the physical, mental, emotional and social dimensions of health.
2. Physical Education – a planned, sequential curriculum that provides learning experiences in a variety of activity areas that all students enjoy and can pursue throughout their lives.
3. Health Services – services provided by health professionals and available to students to appraise, protect and promote health, including counselling and educational opportunities.
4. Nutrition Services – access to a variety of nutritious and appealing meals that accommodate the health and nutritional needs of all students.
5. Counselling and Psychological Services – services provided by professionals to improve students' mental, emotional, and social health.
6. Healthy School Environment – the physical and aesthetic surroundings and the psychosocial climate and culture of the school that affect the well-being of students and staff.
7. Health Promotion for Staff – opportunities for the staff to improve their health status through health assessments, health education and health-related fitness activities.
8. Family–Community Involvement – an integrated school, parent, and community approach for enhancing the health and well-being of students.

The guidelines include and combine two types of strategies: (a) classroom education as an efficient vehicle for health education directed at developing personal health skills and influencing behaviour and health; and (b) a supportive school environment that promotes children's and adolescents' health and social development (Samdal, 2008). Inclusion of the second strategy is a key part of the 'health promoting school' concept. Further, action focused on the environment constitutes the whole school approach, which in all of the networks has been identified as a common core for the health promotion actions. The whole school approach builds on one of the major principles of health promotion, namely collective learning (Kickbusch, 2003). In a school context this may also be seen to parallel organisational learning and change as well as more general educational aims of learning and development. The function of school from an educational and developmental perspective is thus also in focus, highlighting that health promotion contributes more, achieving the school's educational role as well as influencing specific health outcomes.

In many ways the introduction of health promoting schools represented a shift from individual behaviour orientation to a socio-ecological approach, emphasising the interplay between organisations and individuals (Deschesnes, Trudeau & Kébé, 2010; McLeroy, Bibeau, Steckler & Glanz, 1988). The interplay represents an organisational learning process, as change is required at organisational level before expecting change at individual level (Green & Kreuter, 2005). That is, change in organisational structures and processes is employed to achieve change in individual level behaviour and perceptions (Silins, Zarins & Mulford, 2002; Wang & Ahmed, 2003). This interaction also parallels the overall aims of the health promoting school initiative, namely to build supportive contexts to promote individual level health behaviours and perceptions (St Leger, 2000). A prerequisite for the individual change is, however, involvement of the individuals in the organisational change processes. Involvement of students, staff and collaborators such as parents, health professionals and the local community is therefore vital to the success of the process. Furthermore, involving and empowering the target group in the implementation of actions is considered a key principle of health promotion and also specifically meets the basic aims of health promoting schools (Kickbusch, 2003). In building participation three processes are involved. First, involvement equips the participants to become partners. Second, it stimulates learning through that participation. Third, this all contributes to the development process involved in creating health promoting schools.

The strong focus on organisational learning in the health promoting school approach may be seen as a key instigator of the interest taken by the education sector as this matches core development areas in this field (Samdal, 2008; Samdal, et al., 2010). Further, the health promoting schools' focus on developing a psychosocial climate that stimulates students' thriving matches the schools' aims of developing good learning climates. In this process, schools and teachers have been able to utilise their educational theories and practices, and at the same time, work to achieve the aims of the health promoting schools.

The role of the health promoting school networks and associations

A common approach for all the established health promoting school networks has been that they have constituted a vehicle to implement the guidelines through national, regional and local system levels. In the network *Schools for Health in Europe* each country has a national coordinator selected jointly by the Ministry of Education and Ministry of Health. This ministerial anchoring was a requirement for each country's entry to the network and their national work to promote health in school. Still, the fact that the invitation to join the network came from WHO has, in most countries, meant that the health sectors have been the driving force of the health promoting school initiative. For a functional partnership between health and education it is of particular relevance that health sectors understand and acknowledge that health promotion needs to be implemented in line with the objectives of the school. If not, the implementation processes are less beneficial both to the health promotion objectives and the school development in general (Deschesnes, Couturier *et al.*, 2010).

Unlike the European network which was very much established through national top-down approaches, the Australian Health Promoting Schools Association was established as more of a bottom-up approach by health and education professionals, parent groups, non-government organisations and researchers (Rowling, 1996) (see case study, Chapter 7). The national government provided policy and funding for specific projects of national priority. In the 1990s at a national level there was a common philosophy around social justice, reflected in the purpose and process for health and educational outcomes (Hobart Declaration on Schooling, 1989 and National Health Policy, 1994). Individual states through health promotion services had initiated health promoting schools projects. This origin as a project from a health service had a major influence in shaping action, although a number of states did develop joint agreements between education and health sectors.

In Australia, unlike Europe, there was not a dedicated support centre nationally nor a national coordinator, but there was a key policy document, *Effective school health promotion: Towards a health promoting school*, from the peak health body, the National Health and Medical Research Council (NHMRC) (1996). There was also a mandated area of learning health and physical education within a national curriculum framework. The existence of a well developed curriculum was a facilitating factor, providing a supportive context for expansion to include physical and social impacts on school health (Rowling, 1996).

Thus, in both Europe and Australia existing contextual factors influenced the structure and approach of health promoting schools initiatives.

Identification of implementation components

Existing health promoting schools guidelines and indicators have so far not provided sufficiently concrete guidance to schools on quality theory based implementation. Additionally, much of the previous work was reported from a health-based perspective, ignoring the conceptualisation of health promoting schools from an educational research and practice orientation (Deschesnes, Couturier *et al.*, 2010; Mohammadi, Rowling & Nutbeam, 2010; Rowling & Jeffreys, 2006). The guidelines are not enough. Concrete implementation components are needed that take into account the health promoting school objectives to be met, the links with educational outcomes and the context of the implementation process at school and national level. Not only identification of components needs to be given attention, but also their functioning if practitioners are to be able to implement them with fidelity (Dusenbury *et al.*, 2003) and thereby achieve the goals of health promoting schools. Specificity of the components of implementation with concrete/hands-on evidence based actions will help ensure practitioners' understanding and guide their practice. Recording the functioning of the implementation components will further provide a new focus for strengthening the science base for health promoting schools, as has been repeatedly called for over the past decade (Deschesnes, Martin & Hill, 2003; Lister-Sharp, *et al.*, 1999; Stewart-Brown, 2006).

This book thus aims to specify implementation components for health promoting schools and describe their functioning and provide concrete guidance on their application. The empirical delineation of core implementation components will be based on a meta-analysis of the literature. Relevant implementation and organisational change theories will be used to identify the functionality, i.e. the mechanisms at work, for each component. Thereafter concrete guidance on how the mechanisms can be translated and implemented into daily school practice will be provided. As context is a key implementation factor, case studies from varying countries presenting concrete examples of national and local work in a number of countries worldwide are used. These demonstrate global applicability of the implementation components and the different action in different contexts, but with underlying similarities.

The book is structured around three main sections: one addressing the theory base for implementation of health promoting schools, the second providing examples through case studies and the third identifying needs for future developments. Below, each of the parts and their respective chapters are described.

Part I: Theory base for implementation of health promoting schools includes five chapters that articulate the development and main aims of health promoting schools as well as a theory base for implementation, including specific implementation components.

Chapter 1: Introduction has contextualised core principles of health promoting schools, how these relate to school as a learning organisation, and outlined the need for concrete implementation guidelines for health promoting schools.

Chapter 2: Overview of implementation in health promoting settings gives an overview of key implementation issues when health promotion is to be implemented in a setting. Mark Dooris and Margaret Barry detail core principles of settings based implementation of health promotion. Key characteristics of implementation in a school setting and other settings are elucidated.

Chapter 3: Applying system theory of organisational change to health promotion interventions in schools contextualises the health promoting schools within the field of educational change, using systems theory to explain and understand the change process. Wolfgang Dür in this chapter draws on system theory when explaining the complex interactions between individuals and the organisation and how these interactions influence the implementation process.

Chapter 4: Theory based components for implementation of health promoting schools identifies and elaborates on the content and functions of eight implementation components for health promoting schools:

1.   preparing and planning for school development;
2.   policy and institutional anchoring;

3. professional development and learning;
4. leadership and management practices;
5. relational and organisational support context;
6. student participation;
7. partnership and networking;
8. sustainability.

These components have been identified by the editors through a meta-analysis of the literature of implementation studies of health promoting schools. The basis for the components as well as reference to theories and theoretical perspectives that can explain their function are elaborated. Understanding core mechanisms of each component is vital to the effectiveness of implementing health promoting schools. Emphasis is given to building implementation understanding seen from a practitioners' point of view, i.e. teachers, health workers and non-governmental organisations (NGO) participants, as they are the key implementers of health promoting schools.

Chapter 5: Theory based implementation of components builds on Chapter 4, to address the concrete implementation of components. While Chapter 4 covers the content of the components, in Chapter 5 the editors elaborate on how the components are to be implemented by employing implementation theory and empirical findings from the research literature.

Part II: Case studies – *Chapters 6–9* provide concrete examples of implementation approaches in a number of different countries. Each chapter conceptualises and describes implementation within the specific characteristics of their country and structures their text around the components presented in Chapters 4 and 5. Examples are provided from Canada, Europe and Oceania. The countries include Australia, Canada, England, Germany, Norway, Poland, Portugal, and Scotland.

Part III: Conclusions – *Chapter 10: Cross fertilisation of national experiences and need for future developments* highlights how the identified implementation components for health promoting schools can contribute to explaining and understanding the impact of the national and school level activities. In this chapter the editors summarise and identify how the concrete case studies support the hypothesised theoretical assumptions of implementation and system change theories. Furthermore, needs for future developments at practice and research level are identified.

References

Catford, J. (2009). Advancing the 'science of delivery' of health promotion: not just the 'science of discovery'. *Health Promotion International, 24*(1), 1–5.

Clift, S., Bruun-Jensen, B. & Paulus, P. (2005). Introduction. In S. Clift & B. Bruun-Jensen (Eds), *The Health Promoting School: International Advances in Theory, Evaluation and Practice.* Copenhagen: Danish University Press.

Deschesnes, M., Couturier, Y., Laberge, S. & Campeau, L. (2010). How divergent conceptions among health and education stakeholders influence the dissemination of healthy schools in Quebec. *Health Promotion International, 25*(4), 435–443.

Deschesnes, M., Martin, C. & Hill, A. J. (2003). Comprehensive approaches to school health promotion: how to achieve broader implementation? *Health Promotion International, 18*(4), 387–396.

Deschesnes, M., Trudeau, F. & Kébé, M. (2010). Factors influencing the adoption of a Health Promoting School approach in the province of Quebec, Canada. *Health Education Research, 25*(3), 438–450.

Dusenbury, L., Brannigan, R., Falco, M. & Hansen, W. B. (2003). A review of research on fidelity of implementation: implications for drug abuse prevention in school settings. *Health Education Research, 18*(2), 237–256.

ENHPS (1997). *Conference Resolution. First Conference of the European Network of Health Promoting Schools.* Copenhagen: WHO Regional Office for Europe.

Green, L. W. & Kreuter, M. W. (2005). *Health Promotion Planning: An Educational and Ecological Approach* (4th edn). New York, NY: McGraw-Hill.

International Union for Health Promotion and Education (2008). Achieving Health Promoting Schools: Guidelines for Promoting Health in Schools. Retrieved from http://www.iuhpe.org/uploaded/Publications/Books_Reports/HPS_GuidelinesII_2009_English.pdf (accessed 21 September 2012).

International Union for Health Promotion and Education (2009). Promoting Health in Schools: From Evidence to Action. Retrieved from http://www.iuhpe.org/uploaded/Activities/Scientific_Affairs/CDC/PHiS-E&A_3Mar2010_WEB.pdf (accessed 15 March 2012).

Kickbusch, I. (2003). The contribution of the World Health Organization to a new public health and health promotion. *American Journal of Public Health, 93*(3), 383–388.

Leurs, M. T. W., Bessems, K., Schaalma, H. P. & de Vries, H. (2007). Focus points for school health promotion improvements in Dutch primary schools. *Health Education Research, 22*(1), 58–69.

Leurs, M. T. W., Schaalma, H. P., Jansen, M. W. J., Mur-Veeman, I. M., St Leger, L. H. & de Vries, N. (2005). Development of a collaborative model to improve school health promotion in the Netherlands. *Health Promotion International, 20*(3), 296–305.

Lister-Sharp, D., Chapman, S., Stewart-Brown, S. & Sowden, A. (1999). Health promoting schools and health promotion in school: two systematic reviews. *Health Technology Assessment 3*(22), 1–207.

McLeroy, K. R., Bibeau, D., Steckler, A. & Glanz, K. (1988). An ecological perspective on health promotion programs. *Health Education & Behavior, 15*(4), 351–377.

Mohammadi, N. K., Rowling, L. & Nutbeam. (2010). Acknowledging educational perspectives on health promoting schools. *Health Education, 110*(4), 240–251.

National Health and Medical Research Council. (1996). Effective school health promotion: towards health promoting schools. Retrieved from http://www.nhmrc.gov.au/_files_nhmrc/publications/attachments/hp1.pdf (accessed 21 September 2012).

Rowling, L. (1996). The adaptability of the health promoting schools concept: a case study from Australia. *Health Education Research, 11*(4), 519–526.

Rowling L. & Jeffreys, V. (2000). Challenges in the development and monitoring of Health Promoting Schools. *Health Education, 100*, 117–123.

Rowling, L. & Jeffreys, V. (2006). Capturing complexity: integrating health and education research to inform health-promoting schools policy and practice. *Health Education Research, 21*(5), 705–718.

Samdal, O. (2008). School health promotion. In H. Heggenhougen (Ed.), *The Encyclopedia of Public Health* (Vol. 5, pp. 653–661). Oxford: Elsevier Inc.

Samdal, O., Viig, N. G. & Wold, B. (2010). Health promotion integrated into school policy and practice: experiences of implementation in the Norwegian network of health promoting schools. *Journal of Child and Adolescent Psychology, 1*(2), 43–72.

Silins, H., Zarins, S. & Mulford, B. (2002). What characteristics and processes define a school as a learning organisation? Is this a useful concept to apply to schools? *International Education Journal, 3*(1), 24–32.

St Leger, L. (2000). Reducing the barriers to the expansion of health promoting schools by focussing on teachers. *Health Education, 100*(2), 81–87.

Stewart-Brown, S. (2006). What is the evidence on school health promotion in improving health or preventing disease and, specifically, what is the effectiveness of the health promoting schools approach? *Health Evidence Network Report*. Copenhagen: WHO Regional Office for Europe.

Tang, K.-C., Nutbeam, D., Aldinger, C., St Leger, L., Bundy, D., *et al.* (2009). Schools for health, education and development: a call for action. *Health Promotion International, 24*(1), 68–77.

Tjomsland, H. E., Iversen, A. C. & Wold, B. (2009). The Norwegian Network of Health Promoting Schools: A three-year follow-up study of teacher motivation, participation and perceived outcomes. *Scandinavian Journal of Educational Research, 53*(1), 89–102.

Viig, N. G. & Wold, B. (2005). Facilitating Teachers' Participation in School-Based Health Promotion – A Qualitative Study. *Scandinavian Journal of Educational Research, 49*(1), 83–109.

Wang, C. L. & Ahmed, P. K. (2003). Organisational learning: A critical review. *The Learning Organization, 10*(1), 8–17.

Whitelaw S, Baxendale A, Bryce C, MacHardy, L., Young, I. & Witney, E: (2001) Settings' based health promotion: a review, *Health Promotion International*, Vol.16 No. 4, pp. 339–353.

World Health Organization (WHO). (1986). Ottawa Charter for Health Promotion. *Health Promotion International, 1*(4), iii–v.

Young, I. (2005). Health promotion in schools – a historical perspective. *Promotion & Education, 12*(3–4), 1.

Additional websites

www.cdc.gov/HealthyYouth/CSHP/ (accessed 7 October 2010).
www.schoolsforhealt.eu (accessed 10 October 2010).

2

OVERVIEW OF IMPLEMENTATION IN HEALTH PROMOTING SETTINGS

Mark Dooris and Margaret M. Barry

Conceptualising the settings approach to health promotion

The settings approach to health promotion has its roots within the World Health Organization (WHO) Health for All strategy (WHO, 1981) and, specifically, the Ottawa Charter for Health Promotion, which affirmed that: 'Health is created and lived by people within the settings of their everyday life; where they learn, work, play and love' (WHO, 1986). Subsequent global health promotion conferences lent further support and legitimacy to the settings approach. The Sundsvall Statement argued that 'a call for the creation of supportive environments is a practical proposal for public health action at the local level, with a focus on settings for health that allow for broad community involvement and control' (WHO, 1991); the Jakarta Declaration affirmed that 'settings for health represent the organisational base of the infrastructure required for health promotion' and that 'comprehensive approaches to health development are the most effective . . . particular settings offer practical opportunities for the implementation of comprehensive strategies' (WHO, 1997); the Bangkok Charter urged the health sector to work across settings and called on all settings to play a role in advocacy, investment, capacity-building, regulation, legislation and partnership development for health (WHO, 2005); and the Nairobi Call to Action emphasised the importance of intersectoral action and of 'developing political momentum and leadership for health in all policies and settings' (WHO, 2009).

As Kickbusch (1996) has reflected, the Ottawa Charter resulted in the settings approach becoming the starting point for the WHO's lead health promotion programmes, with a commitment to: 'shifting the focus from the deficit model of disease to the health potentials inherent in the social and institutional settings of everyday life . . . [and] pioneer[ing] strategies that strengthened both sense of place and sense of self'. Launched in 1987 by the WHO Regional Office for Europe (Tsouros, 1991), Healthy Cities is widely understood to have been the first settings programme. However, the approach quickly inspired further developments: for example, within Europe, a range of programmes emerged in organisational settings such as schools, universities, hospitals and prisons (Baybutt, Hayton & Dooris, 2006; Pelikan, 2007; Tsouros, Dowding, Thompson & Dooris, 1998; Young, 2005); and elsewhere, a range of programmes were initiated within geographical settings such as districts, communities, islands and marketplaces (Galea, Powis & Tamplin, 2000; O'Neill, Pederson & Rootman, 2000; (WHO, 2002, 2004). The establishment of international settings programmes and networks prepared the way for settings to be included within WHO's Health Promotion Glossary (WHO, 1998a) and incorporated within Regional strategic documents such as Health 21 (WHO, 1998b).

Definition and rationale

It has long been recognised that settings such as schools provide an opportunity to target health messages and interventions. In this way, settings – together with population groups and health topics or problems – make up the traditional matrix used to organise public health programmes focused on individual health-related behaviour change. However, what has become known as the 'settings approach' rejects reductionism – appreciating that many risk and protective factors are interrelated and can be most effectively tackled through comprehensive programmes in settings where people live. Furthermore, it moves beyond targeting only interventions *within* settings, recognising that the culture, ethos and activities of settings are themselves crucially important in determining health and well-being (Dooris *et al.*, 2007; Poland, Krupa & McCall, 2009).

Echoing Wenzel (1997), who viewed settings as spatial, temporal and cultural domains of face-to-face interaction in everyday life that, from the perspective of health promotion, are crucial for the development of lifestyles and living conditions conducive to health, World Health Organization (WHO, 1998a: 19) defined 'settings for health' as: 'The place or social context in which people engage in daily activities in which environmental, organisational and personal factors interact to affect health and well-being . . . where people actively use and shape the environment and thus create or solve problems relating to health. Settings can normally be identified as having physical boundaries, a range of people with defined roles, and an organisational structure.'

Almost a decade ago, Green, Poland & Rootman (2000) drew on critical theory to broaden this conceptualisation and argue against an instrumental view of settings as vehicles for delivering interventions. They also emphasised that most settings are usually oriented to goals other than health and are 'arenas of sustained interaction, with pre-existing structures, policies, characteristics, institutional values, and both formal and informal sanctions on behaviours.'

Recognising that health is largely determined not only by 'health' services and individual lifestyle but also by wider social, economic, environmental, organisational and cultural circumstances, the settings approach represents an investment in the social systems in which people spend their time and live their lives.

A conceptual framework

Although there is, as yet, no overarching 'theory' for healthy settings, Dooris (2006) has proposed a conceptual framework that emphasises the application of underpinning values such as equity, participation, empowerment, partnership and sustainability, and contends that the settings approach has three key characteristics:

- *An ecological model of health promotion:* This reflects a shift of focus from a concern with what makes individuals ill towards a salutogenic perspective (Antonovsky, 1987, 1996) concerned with what creates health in populations. It also represents a move away from a reductionist focus on single issues, risk factors and linear causality towards a more holistic vision that understands health and well-being to be determined by a complex interaction of environmental, organisational and personal factors within the contexts and places where people live their lives.
- *A systems perspective:* Informed by this ecological model and drawing on organisational theory, the approach views settings as complex dynamic systems with inputs, throughputs and outputs (Paton, Sengupta & Hassan, 2005). This perspective acknowledges the value of mapping interconnectedness and synergy between different components, and recognises that settings are both complex and open systems. This implies an appreciation of the connections between different systems and recognition that although organisational development and change can to an extent be planned, it must also allow for unpredictability.
- *Whole system development and change:* The approach uses organisation and/or community development to introduce, manage and sustain change within the setting in its entirety, taking account of contextual norms, values and inter-relationships and applying 'whole system thinking'. Following Barić (1994), the approach is concerned to ensure living and working environments that promote health and productivity; integrate health within the culture, routine life and core business of specific settings; and connect with and improve wider community well-being.

More recently, Poland and colleagues (2009) have presented a framework for use by practitioners to focus attention on and analyse those features of settings that need to be taken into account in designing and delivering sustainable and successful interventions and programmes. It is suggested that this three-part framework (focused on 'understanding settings', 'changing settings' and 'knowledge development and translation') can be used with stakeholders to gain a more sophisticated understanding of the culture, history and unique context within which implementation is taking place – creating opportunities for empowerment and capacity building.

Conceptualising implementation in health promoting settings

The most common definition of implementation is 'how well a proposed programme or intervention is put into practice' (Durlak, 1998), i.e., what the intervention consists of in practice and how it is delivered. From a research perspective, implementation research enhances our ability to map the critical connections between the local context, intervention activities and the intended intermediate and long term outcomes. Understanding the implementation process is, therefore, critical to the effective adoption, replication and dissemination of interventions and facilitates the translation of research into effective practice and the development of practice-based evidence. However, typically, little information is provided in the published research concerning the process and extent of intervention delivery which must occur in order for positive outcomes to be produced. Thus, while the importance of a settings approach to health promotion is increasingly recognised, the development of research and evaluation to inform effective implementation practice in settings has not kept pace (Dooris, 2006; Dooris *et al.*, 2007).

Adopting a settings approach requires a shift in focus away from delivering single discrete interventions and measuring their 'linear' impact on individuals. Implementation and evaluation strategies are needed that will capture the synergistic interaction and impact of multiple interdependent interventions and systems operating at different levels and spheres within the context of specific settings. Inevitably, this is challenging, requiring an appreciation that the process of change is non-linear and involves multiple interdependent systems.

There are, therefore, limitations to the traditional approach to researching the implementation process in settings, due to the methodological challenges involved in capturing complexity and determining the extent of systems change and transformation. Weiner, Lewis, and Linnan (2009) have called for a stronger knowledge and theory base to guide the implementation of complex innovations and interventions in organisational settings. Greenhalgh and colleagues (2005) have also called for development of the following areas: theory driven research, a focus on process rather than 'package', greater emphasis on ecological analyses, a common language, measures and tools, collaboration and coordination, multidisciplinary and multimethod research, meticulous details, and participation between practitioners and researchers. To date, however, health promotion evaluation research has focused largely on initial design and intervention outcomes. There is a relative paucity of data on the quality of implementation necessary for positive outcomes to be produced and sustained.

In the health area more broadly, however, there is an emerging implementation science, which examines the adoption and implementation of evidence-based interventions that are scaled up, also known as Type II translational research (Fixsen, Naoom, Blasé, Friedman & Wallace, 2005). Although there is increasing emphasis on the 'scaling up' and adoption of effective health promotion interventions in the community (Rohrbach, Grana, Sussman & Valente, 2006), little is known about the quality of implementation when interventions are disseminated across diverse cultural and economic settings outside the research context (Gottfredson & Gottfredson, 2002). This calls for a focus on systematically researching the process of implementing interventions in complex naturalistic settings and identifying the factors and conditions, which can facilitate high quality implementation.

Implementation research matters

As Poland and colleagues (2009) observe, a danger of the drive towards evidence-based practice is that local contextual factors that influence the quality of implementation may be given scant consideration. Implementation research is necessary to understand what actually happens during intervention planning and delivery and identify the implications for the quality of interventions as delivered in specific contexts. Implementation information allows for greater understanding of the internal dynamics and operations of interventions, how the intervention components fit together, how the implementers and intervention recipients/users interact and the obstacles they face and resolve in the process. Implementation data are also critical to interpreting positive or negative outcomes as they strengthen any conclusions that can be made about the intervention's role in producing change and inform the replication and maintenance of interventions across settings (Barry, 2007; Barry, Domitrovich & Lara, 2005; Barry & Jenkins, 2007; Durlak, 1998; Greenberg, Domitrovich & Bumbarger, 2001; Micalic, 2002).

If intervention implementation is not monitored and assessed, an outcome evaluation may be assessing an intervention that differs greatly from that originally designed and planned. Without measuring implementation quality, an intervention may be incorrectly judged as ineffective, when in fact negative outcomes occur as a result of poor-quality implementation or shortcomings in the delivery process. This leads to what is known as a Type III error, that is, the intervention as delivered is of such poor quality as to invalidate the outcomes.

Implementation principles

From the existing research a number of implementation principles can be identified. Implementation turns theory and ideas into practice and translates intervention plans into effectively operating programmes (Bracht, Kingsbury & Rissel, 1999). In relation to health promotion interventions this includes adopting an implementation process that is empowering, collaborative, participatory, and carried out in partnership with key stakeholders.

It is clear from research that to assess implementation adequately, information is needed about specific intervention activities or components, how they are delivered, and the characteristics of the context or settings in which the intervention is conducted (Dane & Schneider, 1998). Chen (1998) pointed out that although an intervention is regarded as the major change agent, the 'implementation system' also makes an important contribution to intervention outcomes as it provides the means and the context for the intervention. Therefore, as well as having a clear intervention theory and establishing the essential intervention components that contribute to outcomes, it is necessary to understand the conditions required for successful implementation and the contextual factors that may affect and moderate their effects. Understanding the context and the wider implementation system is, of course, even more critical when implementing a settings approach, as the setting itself constitutes the focus of the intervention. This argument is powerfully reinforced in the context of health promoting settings by Poland and colleagues (2009), whose three-part analytical framework outlined above (and discussed in more detail below) provides a valuable tool to enhance practice.

A conceptual model of the implementation system has been proposed by Chen (1998) and expanded by Greenhalgh and colleagues (2005). It outlines five aspects of implementation which play an integral role in influencing implementation – the characteristic of the implementer (e.g. knowledge, skills and motivation), implementing organisation (e.g. structure, ethos, history, resources), intervention activities (e.g. quality and availability of training, materials etc.) participants (identifying, recruiting, engaging and retaining the target population) and specific context (environment, local policies, agencies and collaborations etc.) that may affect the quality of the intervention implementation and specifically intervention adherence.

Durlak and DuPre (2008) report convergent evidence from a number of systematic reviews (e.g. Fixsen et al., 2005; Greenhalgh et al., 2005; Stith et al., 2006) of the necessity for a multilevel ecological framework for understanding implementation. Building on the work of Chen (1998) and Greenhalgh and colleagues (2005), their review underscores the importance of variables related to the characteristics of the intervention/innovation, the community context of the intervention, the intervention providers, as well as those associated with the intervention delivery and support systems. The review of findings from over 500 studies provides strong empirical support for the conclusion that the level of implementation affects the outcomes obtained and that the multiple ecological factors identified above interact to affect the implementation process. Intervention characteristics reported to be consistently related to implementation are adaptability or flexibility of the intervention and the contextual appropriateness or fit with the organisation. Other important influences identified are the local community politics, funding, policy, and prevention/promotion theory and research. With regard to provider characteristics, Durlak and DuPre (2008) reported that four variables have consistently been found to be related to implementation: perceptions related to the need for, and potential benefits of the intervention, self-efficacy and skill proficiency. Factors related to organisational capacity include general organisational features (e.g. open to change), specific organisational practices and processes (e.g. effective leadership, having at least one programme champion, a collaborative approach, shared decision making), and specific staffing considerations (skills, attitudes, motivations etc.). The delivery system is also found to be critical to effective implementation, including that providers are prepared effectively for their roles, e.g. through development of intervention skills.

The importance of assessing the context specific factors that influence the quality of implementation in the local setting is clearly underscored in the literature, including organisational structures and policies, readiness to implement the intervention both in terms of general organisational capacity and intervention specific capacity, mobilisation of support, and generally determining the ecological fit of the intervention in the local context. Careful delineation and monitoring of the implementation process in settings is needed to provide a clear account of what is actually done (as opposed to planned), how well it is done, influencing factors, and whether the outcomes occur as a result of what was done.

Implementation research is, therefore, critical to understanding intervention strengths and weaknesses, determining how and why interventions work, documenting what actually takes place when an intervention is conducted, and providing feedback for continuous quality improvement in delivery (Domitrovich & Greenberg, 2000).

Implementing complex health promotion interventions

Community settings are intrinsically complex and dynamic, being composed of many sub-settings such as schools, workplaces and neighbourhoods. However, they offer important opportunities to work with diverse population groups across a range of sectors. Complex community interventions are typically composed of multiple intervention components, addressing different population groups, which may be planned to occur across different levels of the social ecology: individual, interpersonal, organisational, community, and macro-policy. Interventions at each level may in turn be logically connected to supportive activities at the next level, i.e. individual skills building linked to supportive community organisation activities. This type of multi-component intervention requires an implementation model, which identifies and maps the sequence of events and their interconnections that are needed for effective outcomes across the various levels.

As previously highlighted, the generation and use of evidence in implementing and sustaining comprehensive health promotion interventions, particularly those adopting a settings approach, is under-researched (Dooris et al., 2007).

However, there are a number of existing models and frameworks for conceptualising implementation. Echoing perspectives highlighted in the literature
conceptualising the settings approach, Poland, Green and Rootman (2000),
Dooris (2006), Greenhalgh, Robert, Macfarlane, Bate and Kyriakidou (2004)
and Fixsen and colleagues (2005) have emphasised the importance of contextual
factors and the complex interaction between individual and organisational factors
and how these in turn interact with the characteristics of the intervention to be
implemented. From an analysis of the existing literature on implementation and
dissemination, Flaspohler, Duffy, Wandersman, Stillman, and Maras (2008)
suggested that different types (individual, organisational, and community) and
levels of capacity (general capacity and innovation-specific capacity) are critical
determinants of effective implementation. Drawing on these various models,
Wandersman and colleagues (2008) outlined an Interactive Systems Framework
(ISF) for Dissemination and Implementation, as a basis for understanding the
key systems, functions and relationships relevant to the implementation and
dissemination process. This framework describes three interacting systems:
Prevention Synthesis and Translation System (distils information about effective
innovations and transfers into user friendly formats); the Prevention Support
System (which provides training, technical assistance and other support to users
and implementers in the field); the Prevention Delivery System (which carries
out the activities necessary to implement interventions in the world of practice).
This Framework, which combines the research-to-practice and community-
centred models of implementation and dissemination, provides a potentially
useful structure for organising theory and research on health promotion implementation. The ISF has particular relevance for implementation in health promotion settings as it focuses on the infrastructure and systems that are needed for
effective implementation to take place and highlights the importance of capacity
within the various systems in a particular setting. Durlak and DuPre (2008)
extended the ISF model to embrace a multilevel ecological framework and
posited that effective implementation is dependent on the favourable interaction
of a constellation of factors operating within these systems (e.g. the intervention/
innovation, providers, communities, prevention delivery system and the prevention support systems) which are specific to the local context. This ecological
model with an emphasis on interacting systems fits well with a settings approach
as the focus is not solely on the implementation of a single discrete intervention
and recognition is given to the broader context within which implementation
takes place.

The analytic framework for implementation proposed by Poland and
colleagues (2009), discussed earlier in this chapter, offers a very useful guide for
undertaking a systematic analysis of a particular setting and its defining characteristics and systems. The framework outlines a series of critical questions for the
analysis of settings, which could be used to develop an ecological logic model of
how the intervention process addresses the localised determinants of health in
the specific setting, including how the setting itself can be transformed to become

more health promoting. The capacity of the setting for change needs to be determined, including structural and organisational change, so that the implementation process addresses change in the setting itself as well as change for the people to be found in the setting. This framework provides a useful template for systematically analysing and documenting the critical features of settings, which can impact on intervention design and implementation.

Implementation in school settings

Taking the school setting as an example, schools are dynamic multi-level systems with numerous factors that can influence implementation (Barry *et al.*, 2005; Durlak, 1998; Elias, Bruene-Butler, Blum & Schuyler, 2000; Gottfredson, Fink, Skroban & Gottfredson, 1997; Hoagwood & Johnson, 2003; Mihalic, 2002; Weissberg & Greenberg, 1998).

To date, the systematic study of intervention implementation in the whole school setting has been relatively neglected. However, from the research conducted to date it is clear that implementation represents a complex interaction between characteristics of the implementation system, characteristics of the implementer, and various aspects of the setting and organisational context in which the intervention is implemented (Chen, 1998; Dariotis, Bumbarger, Duncan & Greenberg, 2008; Greenberg *et al.*, 2006).

As highlighted earlier in this chapter, Durlak and DuPre (2008) reported persuasive evidence of the powerful impact of quality of implementation on outcomes, including in school-based interventions. Regarding the interactions among contextual factors, a small number of studies have assessed the relative influence of different factors on implementation in school settings. Kallestad and Olweus (2003) found that the effective implementation of school-wide anti-bullying programmes in Norway is predicted by both individual and school level variables such as teachers' perception of the problem, school climate, and leadership in the school setting on anti-bullying. Kam, Greenberg, and Walls (2003) also reported a significant interaction between level of principal support and the fidelity of teachers' implementation on student outcomes in school-based mental health programmes. With regard to the whole school approach, implementation studies assessing the influence of variables operating across the different ecological levels in the whole school setting (individual, organisational and community levels) are, therefore, needed to understand the interactions that may occur among contextual factors in the local setting.

Understanding the community, organisational and cultural contexts of schools is critical for implementation and sustainability of interventions because children, teachers and other school staff are all embedded in this shared environment (Bumbarger, Perkins & Greenberg, in press; Ringeisen, Henderson & Hoagwood, 2003). Research on organisational factors has shown that implementation is more likely to be successful in organisations that have strong administration, leadership, and support for the intervention (Farrell, Meyer, Kung & Sullivan,

2001; Kam, *et al.*, 2003; Kegler, Steckler, Malek & McLeroy, 1998; Rohrbach, Graham & Hansen, 1993), stability in terms of resources and personnel, and also communication patterns that are open and clear (Domitrovich *et al.*, 2008; Gottfredson & Gottfredson, 2002; Kegler, *et al.*, 1998; Rohrbach, *et al.*, 2006). Another important organisational practice supporting implementation in several studies is shared decision making, i.e., collaboration with and involvement of community members, support of parents, local input and local ownership (Durlak & DuPre, 2008).

At the level of characteristics of the implementer, the knowledge, skills, and motivation of the programme implementer play a significant role in successful programme implementation. The perceptions of teachers related to the intervention, their self-efficacy and skill proficiency have been found to promote or undermine implementation in schools (Domitrovich, *et al.*, 2008). As outlined earlier, all of these factors interact with characteristics of the intervention (such as its ecological fit with the school) and the intervention delivery and support systems, including training, technical assistance and support for implementers.

Factors in the whole school context are, therefore, critical for successful implementation. The whole school context includes the school's environment and ethos, organisation, management structures, relationships with parents and the wider community as well as the taught curriculum and pedagogic practice (Weare, 2000). Evidence from systematic reviews supports the effectiveness of universal health promotion programmes in schools that take a whole school approach involving staff and students, the wider school environment and local community (Lister-Sharp *et al.*, 1999; Stewart-Brown, 2006; Wells, Barlow & Stewart-Brown, 2003). Understanding the complex interaction of influencing factors within a whole school context, therefore, plays a vital role in determining quality of implementation and hence overall effectiveness.

The specific context of disadvantaged schools in Ireland participating in an international emotional well-being programme for primary school children was reported by Clarke, O'Sullivan, and Barry (2010). Within the framework of the overall evaluation study, which employed a cluster randomis\ed controlled design, case studies were employed. It provided an insight into the contextual factors impacting on programme implementation in disadvantaged school settings. The case study method explored the views of teachers, pupils, parents and key informants from the wider community on the delivery of the programme within the context of a whole school approach. The findings are from two contrasting schools, a large urban school with a multi-cultural profile in an area of multiple disadvantage and a smaller, almost monocultural, rural school in the border region with Northern Ireland. With regard to the community context of the schools, the data indicated contrasting levels of community engagement and parental involvement in the two schools. The perceived lack of a cohesive community context and low levels of parental involvement in the large urban school contributed to a more challenging environment for programme implementation. Perceived community context variables are predictive of teacher–parent relationships (Wandersmen *et al.*, 2007) and teachers may not fully appreciate the impact of social and economic factors on parent involvement. These findings underscore the importance of socio–economic and cultural influences in the local communities and the challenges they present for effective implementation. In relation to organisational practices and processes, differences emerged between the teachers in the two schools regarding the perceived school ethos and environment, particularly with regard to school practices in supporting children during stressful periods and developing positive open relationships between staff, children and parents.

Concerning characteristics of the implementers, despite similar levels of reported implementation fidelity, the teachers in the small rural school had a much more positive view of the programme and reported positive programme influences on the classroom atmosphere and on their own capacity to help the children. These results were not evident from the urban school where teachers' attitudes were much less positive.

The case study highlighted the uniqueness of both schools with their differing community histories, cultures, local politics and organisational capacity and structures. The capacity development needs of both schools are quite different, particularly with regard to community and parental involvement. In relation to the teachers, it was evident that those in the large urban school were less positive about the programme. Although both schools received the same level of training and support, stronger links with local support agencies and staff were reported by the rural school. The less positive attitudes of the teachers in the urban school would suggest the need for on-going technical assistance and support in addressing perceived barriers to effective implementation.

The case study findings indicated that the two schools were at very different stages of 'readiness' in terms of implementing the intervention within a whole school context. The findings point to the important influence of contextual factors on programme implementation in disadvantaged school settings, including characteristics of the local community context, level of parental involvement, school ethos and practices, and teachers' attitudes to the intervention. Therefore, strategies for school organisational change to support implementation would need to be adapted for each school. The findings revealed that many of the factors which affect programme implementation, such as levels of parental involvement, school ethos and policies, community histories, local politics etc., are whole school practices whose particular combinations create a unique school culture within which programme implementation occurs. These findings, which are in keeping with the implementation research to date, indicate the need for evaluation approaches to include assessment and monitoring of the complex interaction of factors operating at the classroom, school, and wider community level that impact on implementation.

As this study and others have illustrated, the systematic collection of data on implementation plays an essential role in interpreting intervention outcomes and in advancing knowledge on practice-based evidence (Barry & Jenkins, 2007).

More detailed research on the implementation process is needed in order to provide a deeper understanding of the contextual factors impacting on implementation, thereby facilitating better implementation and more effective capacity building for sustainable change at a whole school level.

Evaluating the effectiveness of a settings approach: challenges and reflections

Dooris and colleagues (2007) conclude that despite the perceived added value of the settings approach and significant advances in evaluation, there is still an 'uneven and under-developed evidence base' (p. 335). In the words of St Leger over a decade ago (St Leger, 1997: 100), 'the settings approach has been legitimated more through an act of faith than through rigorous research and evaluation studies . . . much more attention needs to be given to building the evidence and learning from it.'

The challenges inherent in building a sound evidence base for health promotion are, of course, not unique to settings interventions. As Nutbeam (1999: 99) has commented: 'It is a challenge to assemble "evidence" in ways which are relevant to the complexities of contemporary health promotion, and to avoid the possibility that this may lead action down a narrow, reductionist route.' In response to this challenge, there has been an increased focus on multi-method evaluation, on developing an 'evidence into practice into evidence' cycle, and on generating understanding not only of what works, but also of how, why and when. However, those using the settings approach face three additional challenges (Dooris, 2006; Dooris *et al.*, 2007):

1 Diversity of conceptual understandings and real-life practice

There is a wide range of both understanding and real-life practice incorporated under the settings 'banner' (Poland, *et al.*, 2000; Whitelaw *et al.*, 2001) – one important consequence of which is the difficulty of comparability and transferability within research and evaluation. This reflects a lack of conceptual precision; the application of the approach within and across a multitude of organisational, place-based and informal settings, diverse in size and form; the difficulty of translating theory into practice and the influence of particular implementation contexts; and the conflation of 'health promotion in settings' with the settings approach.

2 Construction of the evidence base: focus on diseases and single risk factors

The primary focus of most systematic reviews, meta-analyses and resulting guidance has tended to be single risk factor interventions and specific diseases and problems, rather than multiple interventions and settings. A limited number of reviews have explicitly considered interventions such as health promoting schools (e.g. Lister-Sharp *et al.*, 1999; Stewart-Brown, 2006) and drawn promising conclusions regarding the value of a whole system approach. Despite this, most reviews that consider a particular setting are concerned to assess the value of discrete interventions.

It would, then, appear that irrespective of discussion of a 'paradigm shift' in health promotion (Barić, 1994) nearly two decades ago, the evidence base has continued to be informed largely by a traditional experimental approach more akin to that applied in the medical model. This reflects the continuing priority given to behaviour and disease-based targets in health policy (Ziglio, Hagard & Griffiths, 2000), leading to more funding being available for evaluation of issue-based than settings initiatives. Consequently, most research designed to evaluate complex, ecological interventions struggles to meet inclusion criteria for systematic reviews – although there is a degree of optimism that this is changing (Jackson & Waters, 2005) as reflected in more recent guidelines (Armstrong *et al.*, 2007).

3 Complexity of evaluating ecological whole system approaches

As highlighted previously, a settings approach is characterised by an ecological model, a systems perspective and whole system thinking. Evaluation, therefore, involves addressing the overall ethos and culture of a particular setting, implementing multiple interrelated interventions adapted to its specific needs, and prioritising organisation development and community empowerment approaches to ensure wide-ranging stakeholder ownership. The reality is, the task of evaluating the settings approach is very complex – due to its systemic nature and its focus on integrating health and well-being into the routine life of settings.

As illustrated in Figure 2.1, the settings approach focuses on the interactions and interdependence of different elements within the complex system, requiring a focus not only on the individual components but on the spaces in-between, on the arrows that join up the boxes in addition to the boxes themselves (Barić & Barić, 1995). Taking health promoting schools as its focus, this diagram identifies organisational context, implementer characteristics, intervention delivery and community context as the core components, within which a range of interconnected influencing factors are nested. Rowling and Jeffreys (2006) comment that: 'Researchers fail to recognize and monitor the synergy created by integrating components, give it minor status in reporting or omit "process" completely. This ignores an essential quality in a settings approach – the interaction of components in a specific context.' The importance of appreciating the synergy between settings adds further complexity to the evaluation challenge, and highlights the value of adopting a coordinated approach (Dooris, 2004).

The concern of the settings approach to move beyond the implementation of interventions to embed effective action for health and well-being within core

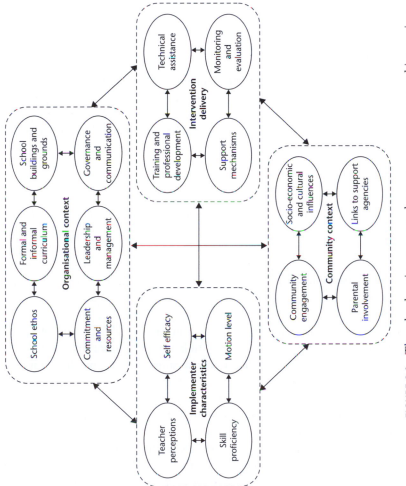

FIGURE 2.1 The school setting as a complex system: components and interactions

business means that, paradoxically, the more successful a settings programme is, the harder it will be to isolate its unique contribution to change at organisational, community and individual levels. Integrative approaches allow the language of 'health' to move to the background – and as the work becomes mainstreamed, 'health promotion' as a discrete entity becomes more distant. A review of workplace health promotion illustrates this, concluding that many organisation-level interventions are 'performed without any direct link to health and thus have an unspecified effect on ill health and well-being' (Breuker and Schröer, 2000: 103–104).

Conclusions

In exploring the implications of these challenges for future research, Dooris and colleagues (2007) reflected that while there has been a growing recognition of the importance of ecology and systems thinking in health promotion (Green, Richard & Potvin, 1996; Stokols, 1996), this has not resulted in clear guidance to inform research and evaluation. In looking to the future, two points can be usefully highlighted:

First, it will be necessary to strengthen and further develop theory (Dooris, 2006) in order to support policy and practice, but also to inform evaluative research and ensure that it is able to help build evidence of effectiveness. There is a growing literature on theory based evaluation and its use in relation to complex initiatives (e.g. Birckmayer & Weiss, 2000; de Leeuw & Skovgaard, 2005) and a call for stronger engagement with critical realism and realist evaluation – which, it is argued, offers the potential 'to "unpack the mechanism" of how complex programmes work (or why they fail) in particular contexts and settings' (Pawson *et al*, 2004: 1).

Second, it seems clear that in order to capture the added value of settings programmes, we must design evaluation studies that do more than focus on the implementation of seemingly disconnected interventions in the context of settings. Instead, we must adopt non-linear approaches, looking at the whole and mapping and elucidating the inter-relationships, interactions and synergies within and between settings – with regard to different components of the system, different issues and different groups of people (Dooris, 2006). This means moving beyond conventional evaluation approaches that are both linear and reductionist, and engaging with complexity theory – which places more emphasis on the organic, emergent nature of innovation and adaptation, and suggests different principles for the management of organisational and social change initiatives (Keshavarz, Nutbeam, Rowling & Khavarpour, 2010). In so doing, it will be important to integrate 'health' measures with measures relating to the core business of the setting (Lee, Cheng & St Leger, 2005; Rowling & Jeffreys, 2006); use multi-method approaches (Pan American Health Organisation, 2005); and recognise the synergistic effects of combining methods to answer a range of evaluation questions (Baum, 1995; Steckler *et al.*, 1992).

References

Antonovsky, A. (1987). *Unraveling the Mystery of Health. How People Manage Stress and Stay Well.* San Francisco, CA: Jossey-Bass Inc.

Antonovsky, A. (1996). The salutogenic model as a theory to guide health promotion. *Health Promotion International, 11*(1), 11–18.

Armstrong, R., Waters, E., Jackson, N., Oliver, S., Popay, J., Shepherd, J., *et al.* (2007). *Guidelines for Systematic Reviews of Health Promotion and Public Health Interventions.* Melbourne: Melbourne University.

Barić, L. (1994). *Health Promotion and Health Education in Practice. Module 2: The Organisational Model.* Altrincham: Barns Publications.

Barić, L. & Barić, L. (1995). *Health Promotion and Health Education. Module 3: Evaluation, Quality, Audit.* Altrincham: Barns Publications.

Barry, M. M. (2007). Building capacity for effective implementation of mental health promotion. *e-Journal for the Advancement of Mental Health, 6*(2), 1–9.

Barry, M. M., Domitrovich, C. E. & Lara, M. A. (2005). The implementation of mental health promotion programme. *Promotion & Education, 2*, 30–36.

Barry, M. M. & Jenkins, R. (2007). *Implementing Mental Health Promotion.* Oxford: Churchill Livingstone/Elsevier.

Baum, F. (1995). Researching public health: beyond the qualitative and quantitative method debate. *Social Science and Medicine, 55*, 459–468.

Baybutt, M., Hayton, P. & Dooris, M. (2006). Prisons in England and Wales: an important public health opportunity? In J. Douglas, S. Earle, S. Handsley, C. Lloyd & S. Spurr (Eds), *Reader in Promoting Public Health: Challenge and Controversy.* London/ Milton Keynes: Sage/Open University Press.

Birckmayer, J. & Weiss, C. (2000). Theory-based evaluation in practice. What do we learn? *Evaluation Review, 24*, 407–431.

Bracht, N., Kingsbury, L. & Rissel, C. (1999). A five-stage community organization model for health promotion: empowerment and partnership strategies. In N. Bracht (Ed.), *Health Promotion at the Community Level 2: New Advances* (pp. 83–117). Newbury Park, CA, California: Sage.

Breuker, G. & Schröer, A. (2000) Settings 1 – health promotion in the workplace. In International Union for Health Promotion and Education, *The Evidence of Health Promotion Effectiveness. Shaping Public Health in a New Europe.* Part Two: Evidence Book. ECSC-EC-EAEC, Brussels.

Bumbarger, B. K., Perkins, D. F. & Greenberg, M. T. (In Press). Taking effective prevention to scale. In B. Doll, W. Pfohl & J. Yoon (Eds), *Handbook of Youth Prevention Science.* New York: Routledge.

Chen, H. (1998). Theory-drive evaluations. *Advances in Educational Productivity, 7*, 15–34.

Clarke, A., O'Sullivan, M. & Barry, M. M. (2010). Context matters in programme implementation *Health Education, 110*(4), 273–293.

Dane, A. V. & Schneider, B. H. (1998). Program integrity in primary and early secondary prevention: are implementation effects out of control? *Clinical Psychology Review, 18*(1), 23–45.

Dariotis, J. K., Bumbarger, B. K., Duncan, L. G. & Greenberg, M. T. (2008). How do implementation efforts relate to program adherence? Examining the role of organizational, implementer, and program factors. *Journal of Community Psychology, 36*(6), 744–760.

de Leeuw, E. & Skovgaard, T. (2005). Utility-driven evidence for healthy cities: Problems with evidence generation and application. *Social Science & Medicine, 61*(6), 1331–1341.

Domitrovich, C. E., Bradshaw, C. P., Poduska, J. M., Hoagwood, K., Buckley, J. A., Olin, S., *et al.* (2008). Maximizing the implementation quality of evidence-based preventive interventions in schools: a conceptual framework. *Advances in School Mental Health Promotion*, *1*(3), 6–28.

Domitrovich, C. E. & Greenberg, M. T. (2000). The study of implementation: current findings from effective programs that prevent mental disorders in school-aged children. *Journal of Educational and Psychological Consultation*, *11*(2), 193–221.

Dooris, M. (2004) Joining up settings for health: a valuable investment for strategic partnerships? *Critical Public Health*, *14*, 37–49.

Dooris, M. (2006). Healthy settings: challenges to generating evidence of effectiveness. *Health Promotion International*, *21*(1), 55–65.

Dooris, M., Poland, B., Kolbe, L., de Leeuw, E., McCall, D. & Wharf-Higgins, J. (2007). Healthy settings: building evidence for the effectiveness of whole system health promotion – challenges and future directions. In D. V. McQueen & C. M. Jones (Eds), *Global Perspectives on Health Promotion Effectiveness*. New York: Springer Science and Business Media.

Durlak, J. A. (1998). Why Program Implementation is Important. *Journal of Prevention & Intervention in the Community*, *17*(2), 5–18.

Durlak, J. A. & DuPre, E. (2008). Implementation matters: a review of research on the influence of implementation on program outcomes and the factors affecting implementation. *American Journal of Community Psychology*, *41*(3), 327–350.

Elias, M. J., Bruene-Butler, L., Blum, L. & Schuyler, T. (2000). Voices from the field: identifying and overcoming roadblocks to carrying out programs in social and emotional learning/emotional intelligence. *Journal of Educational and Psychological Consultation*, *11*(2), 253–272.

Farrell, A. D., Meyer, A. L., Kung, E. M. & Sullivan, T. N. (2001). Development and evaluation of school-based violence prevention programs. *Journal of Clinical Child & Adolescent Psychology*, *30*(2), 207–220.

Fixsen, D. L., Naoom, S. F., Blasé, K. A., Friedman, R. M. & Wallace, F. (2005). *Implementation Research: A Synthesis of the Literature*. Tampa, FL: University of South Florida.

Flaspohler, P., Duffy, J., Wandersman, A., Stillman, L. & Maras, M. (2008). Unpacking prevention capacity: an intersection of research-to-practice models and community-centered models. *American Journal of Community Psychology*, *41*(3), 182–196.

Galea, G., Powis, B. & Tamplin, S. A. (2000). Healthy islands in the Western Pacific – international settings development. *Health Promotion International*, *15*(2), 169–178.

Gottfredson, D. C., Fink, C. M., Skroban, S. B. & Gottfredson, G. D. (1997). Making prevention work. In R. P. Weissberg, T. P. Gullotta, R. L. Hampton, B. A. Ryan & G. R. Adams (Eds), *Healthy Children 2010: Establishing Preventive Services* (pp. 219–252). Thousand Oaks, CA: Sage.

Gottfredson, D. C. & Gottfredson, G. D. (2002). Quality of School-Based Prevention Programs: Results from a National Survey. *Journal of Research in Crime and Delinquency*, *39*(1), 3–35.

Green, L., Poland, B. & Rootman, I. (2000). 'The Settings Approach to Health Promotion'. In B. Poland, L. Green & I. Rootman (Eds), *Settings for Health Promotion: Linking Theory and Practice* (pp 1–43). London: Sage.

Green, L. W., Richard, L. & Potvin, L. (1996). Ecological foundations of health promotion. *American Journal of Health Promotion*, *10*(4), 270–281.

Greenberg, M. T., Domitrovich, C. E. & Bumbarger, B. K. (2001). The prevention of mental disorders in school-aged children: Current state of the field. *Prevention & Treatment*, *4*(1), 1–52.

Greenberg, M. T., Weissberg, R., O'Brien, M., Zins, J., Fredericks, L., Resnik, H. & Elias, M. J. (2003). Enhancing school-based prevention and youth development through coordinated social, emotional, and academic learning. *American Psychologist*, *58*(6/7), 466–474.

Greenberg, M. T., Domitrovich, C. E., Graczyk, P. A. & Zins, J. E. (2006). *The Study of Implementation in School-Based Prevention Research: Implications for Theory, Research, and Practice*. Rockville, MD: Centre for Mental Health Services, Substance Abuse and Mental Health Services Administration.

Greenhalgh, T., Robert, G., Bate, P., Kyrakidou, O., Macfarlane, F. & Peacock, R. (2005). *Diffusion of Innovations in Health Service Organisations: A Systematic Literature Review*. Oxford: Blackwell Publishing.

Greenhalgh, T., Robert, G., Macfarlane, F., Bate, P. & Kyriakidou, O. (2004). Diffusion of innovations in service organizations: systematic review and recommendations. *Milbank Quarterly*, *82*(4), 581–629.

Hoagwood, K. & Johnson, J. (2003). School psychology: A public health framework. I. From evidence-based practices to evidence-based policies. *Journal of School Psychology*, *41*(1), 3–21.

Jackson, N. & Waters, E. (2005). *Guidelines: Systematic Reviews of Health Promotion and Public Health Interventions*. Melbourne: Cochrane Collaboration – Cochrane Health Promotion and Public Health Field.

Kallestad, J. H. & Olweus, D. (2003). Predicting teachers' and schools' implementation of the Olweus bullying prevention program: A multilevel study. *Prevention & Treatment*, *6*(1), Article 21.

Kam, C.-M., Greenberg, M. T. & Walls, C. T. (2003). Examining the role of implementation quality in school-based prevention using the PATHS curriculum. *Prevention Science*, *4*(1), 55–63.

Kegler, M. C., Steckler, A., Malek, S. H. & McLeroy, K. (1998). A multiple case study of implementation in 10 local Project ASSIST coalitions in North Carolina. *Health Education Research*, *13*(2), 225–238.

Keshavarz, N., Nutbeam, D., Rowling, L. & Khavarpour, F. (2010). Schools as social complex adaptive systems: A new way to understand the challenges of introducing the health promoting schools concept. *Social Science & Medicine*, *70*(10), 1467–1474.

Kickbusch, I. (1996). Tribute to Aaron Antonovsky – 'What creates health'. *Health Promotion International*, *11*(1), 5–6.

Lee, A., Cheng, F. F. K. & St Leger, L. (2005). Evaluating health-promoting schools in Hong Kong: development of a framework. *Health Promotion International*, *20*(2), 177–186.

Lister-Sharp, D., Chapman, S., Stewart-Brown, S. & Sowden, A. (1999). Health promoting schools and health promotion in school: two systematic reviews. *Health Technology Assessment*, *3*(22), 1–207.

Mihalic, S. (2002). *The importance of implementation fidelity*. Boulder, CO: Center for the Study and Prevention of Violence.

Nutbeam, D. (1999). The challenge to provide 'evidence' in health promotion. *Health Promotion International*, *14*(2), 99–101.

O'Neill, M., Pederson, A. & Rootman, I. (2000). Health promotion in Canada: declining or transforming? *Health Promotion International*, *15*(2), 135–141.

Paton, K., Sengupta, S. & Hassan, L. (2005). Settings, systems and organization development: the Healthy Living and Working model. *Health Promotion International, 20*(1), 81–89.

Pawson, R., Greenhalgh, T., Harvey, G. & Walshe, K. (2004). Realist synthesis: An introduction. ESRC Research Methods Programme (Working Paper Series) (Vol. RMP Methods Paper 2/2004). Manchester: University of Manchester.

Pelikan, J. (2007). Health promoting hospitals – assessing developments in the network. *Italian Journal of Public Health, 4,* 261–270.

Poland, B., Green, L. & Rootman, I. (2000). *Settings for Health Promotion: Linking Theory and Practice.* London: Sage.

Poland, B., Krupa, G. & McCall, D. (2009). Settings for health promotion: an analytic framework to guide intervention design and implementation. *Health Promotion Practice, 10*(4), 505–516.

Ringeisen, H., Henderson, K. & Hoagwood, K. (2003). Context matters: Schools and the "research to practice gap" in children's mental health. *School Psychology Review, 32*(2), 153–168.

Rohrbach, L. A., Graham, J. W. & Hansen, W. B. (1993). Diffusion of a school-based substance abuse prevention program: predictors of program implementation. *Preventive Medicine, 22*(2), 237–260.

Rohrbach, L. A., Grana, R., Sussman, S. & Valente, T. W. (2006). Type II Translation. *Evaluation & the Health Professions, 29*(3), 302–333.

Rowling, L. & Jeffreys, V. (2006). Capturing complexity: integrating health and education research to inform health-promoting schools policy and practice. *Health Education Research, 21*(5), 705–718.

St Leger, L. (1997). Editorial. Health promoting settings: form Ottawa to Jakarta. *Health Promotion International, 12*(2), 99–101.

Steckler, A., McLeroy, K., Goodman, R. M., Bird, S. T. and McCormick L. (1992). Towards integrating qualitative and quantitative methods: an introduction. *Health Education Quarterly, 19*(1–8).

Stewart-Brown, S. (2006). What is the evidence on school health promotion in improving health or preventing disease and, specifically, what is the effectiveness of the health promoting schools approach? *Health Evidence Network Report.* Copenhagen: WHO Regional Office for Europe.

Stith, S., Pruitt, I., Dees, J., Fronce, M., Green, N., Som, A. & Linkh, D. (2006). Implementing community-based prevention programming: a review of the literature. *The Journal of Primary Prevention, 27*(6), 599–617.

Stokols, D. (1996). Translating social ecological theory into guidelines for community health promotion. *American Journal of Health Promotion, 10*(4), 282–298.

Tsouros, A. (1991). *World Health Organization Healthy Cities Project: A Project Becomes a Movement. Review of Progress 1987–1990.* Milan: Sogess.

Tsouros, A., Dowding, G., Thompson, J. & Dooris, M. (1998). *Health Promoting Universities: Concept, Experience and Framework for Action.* Copenhagen: WHO Regional Office for Europe.

Wandersman, A., Duffy, J., Flaspohler, P., Noonan, R., Lubell, K., Stillman, L., *et al.* (2008). Bridging the gap between prevention research and practice: the interactive systems framework for dissemination and implementation. *American Journal of Community Psychology, 41*(3), 171–181.

Weare, K. (2000). *Promoting Mental, Emotional and Social Health: A Whole School Approach.* London: Routledge.

Weiner, B. J., Lewis, M. A. & Linnan, L. A. (2009). Using organization theory to understand the determinants of effective implementation of worksite health promotion programs. *Health Education Research*, *24*(2), 292–305.

Weissberg, R. P. & Greenberg, M. T. (1998). School and community competence-enhancement and prevention programs. In W. Damon, I. E. Sigel & K. A. Renninger (Eds), *Handbook of Child Psychology: Vol 4. Child Psychology in Practice* (5th edn, pp. 877–954). New York: John Wiley & Sons.

Wells, J., Barlow, J. & Stewart-Brown, S. (2003). A systematic review of universal approaches to mental health promotion in schools. *Health Education*, *103*(4), 197–220.

Wenzel, E. (1997). A comment on settings in health promotion. *Internet Journal of Health Promotion*. Retrieved from http: //rhpeo.net/ijhp-articles/1997/1/index.htm (accessed 21 September 2012).

Whitelaw, S., Baxendale, A., Bryce, C., MacHardy, L., Young, I. & Witney, E. (2001). 'Settings' based health promotion: a review. *Health Promotion International*, *16*(4), 339–353.

World Health Organization (WHO) (1981). *Global Strategy for Health for All by the Year 2000*. Geneva: WHO.

World Health Organization (WHO) (1986). *The Ottawa Charter for Health Promotion*. Copenhagen: WHO Regional Office for Europe.

World Health Organization (WHO) (1991). *Sundsvall Statement on Supportive Environments for Health*. Copenhagen: WHO Regional Office for Europe.

World Health Organization (WHO) (1997). *Jakarta Declaration on Health Promotion into the 21st Century*. Geneva: WHO.

World Health Organization (WHO) (1998a). *Health Promotion Glossary*. Geneva: WHO.

World Health Organization (WHO) (1998b). *The Health for All Policy for the WHO European Region – 21 Targets for the 21st Century*. Copenhagen: WHO Regional Office for Europe.

World Health Organization (WHO) (2002). *Integrated Management of Healthy Settings at the District Level. Report of an Intercountry Consultation*. New Delhi: WHO Regional Office for South-East Asia.

World Health Organization (WHO) (2004). *Healthy Marketplaces in the Western Pacific: Guiding Future Action. Applying a Settings Approach to the Promotion of Health in Marketplaces*. Manila: WHO Regional Office for the Western Pacific.

World Health Organization (WHO) (2005). *Bangkok Charter for Health Promotion in a Globalized World*. Geneva: WHO.

World Health Organization (WHO) (2009). *Nairobi Call to Action for Closing the Implementation Gap in Health Promotion*. Geneva: WHO.

Young, I. (2005). Health promotion in schools – a historical perspective. *Promotion & Education*, *12*(3–4), 112–117.

Ziglio, E., Hagard, S. & Griffiths, J. (2000). Health promotion development in Europe: achievements and challenges. *Health Promotion International*, *15*(2), 143–154.

3

APPLYING SYSTEM THEORY OF ORGANISATIONAL CHANGE TO HEALTH PROMOTION INTERVENTIONS IN SCHOOLS[1]

Wolfgang Dür

Background

In most developed countries, schools have become the focus of public criticism. The PISA and TIMSS studies (International Association for the Evaluation of Educational Achievement, 2008; OECD, 2010a, 2010b, 2010c) alerted the public to the problems by pointing to the ineffectiveness and inefficiency of schools and school systems: that after eight or nine years of schooling, there is still a considerable percentage of young people who cannot read or calculate or master even simple problem solving tasks. These studies have also shown that a country's prosperity is not a prerequisite for good educational outcomes. In fact, countries of similar prosperity can produce very different educational results, and low national income is not at all incompatible with strong educational performance (OECD, 2010c).

Complaints come from the economic sectors in society, about the lack of capacities regarding challenges of postmodern life, and working conditions such as self-competence, social and communicational competences, creativity, and innovation orientation.

Additionally the international HBSC study (Currie *et al.*, 2008) has revealed that schools must be seen as a precarious area in terms of health and well-being of their students, and also of their staff (e.g. Bricheno, Brown & Lubansky, 2009; Due *et al.*, 2003; Rasmussen, Mogens, Holstein, Poulsen & Due, 2005; Ravens-Sieberer, Freeman, Kokonyei, Thomas & Erhart, 2009; Samdal, Wold, Klepp & Kannas, 2000; Torsheim & Wold, 2001).

Consequently in nearly all OECD countries, efforts are being made and intensified to further develop schools as the central organisation of modern education systems (OECD, 2010b, 2010c). The scientific groundings of such efforts stem from psychology, sociology, education science, pedagogy, neuroscience, or learning theory, which all reproduce their specific disciplinary perspectives and, within the disciplines, different schools of thinking. As a consequence, none of these scientific discourses, and even less their combination, offer a solid ground for clear straightforward goals and strategies for changes in education politics and in school management – at least not solid enough to lead to a strong consensus among those affected. In this controversial situation, two discourses that avoid disciplinary and ideological conflicts have made their way into school development: health promotion and quality management.

Health promotion and quality management

Health promotion in the settings approach (World Health Organization (WHO), 1986) aims not only at behaviour changes of individuals, but also at improvements regarding structures, processes and environments of organisations which, as a whole, are seen to be the containments of relevant health determinants. Health promotion, therefore, is an instrument of quality improvement with a broad range of applications. As for schools, this range is summarised by the so-called whole school approach (e.g. Deschesnes, Martin & Hill, 2003; Hargreaves, 2008; St Leger, Young, Blanchard & Perry, 2010), that encourages schools to develop complex change projects with a holistic view of their favourable and unfavourable circumstances, even involving the closer community, like parents, and including teaching and learning processes and the school climate.

Today, after two decades of experience, it can be stated that school health promotion has proven to be a useful instrument of school development, through comprehensive, multifactorial, and intense change projects of long duration and at organisational level (Mukoma & Flisher, 2004; Stewart-Brown, 2006).

However, this type of project is difficult to develop and rather complex and challenging when it comes to implementation. Hardly any of the schools involved in those evaluation projects that Stewart-Brown included in her meta-study (Stewart-Brown, 2006) adopted all of the principles of the so-called health promoting school or whole school approach as defined by the WHO. There are indications that many schools, although committed to the concept, feel unable to master its challenges, which demand high skills in management theory and techniques. Principal and teacher in-service training, is therefore, claimed to be a prerequisite for the successful implementation of health promotion (Flaschberger, Nitsch & Waldherr, 2012; St Leger, *et al.*, 2010).

Since the late 1980s, quality management has been widely spread over enterprises and firms. Of course, this was a reaction to new dynamics in the whole economic system and to the demanded flexibility that forced enterprises to have access to effective tools for quick adaptations. Consequently, quality management and especially its basic tool, the so-called PDCA-cycle[2] (Deming, 1986) which instructs the implementation of any strategic decision into an enterprise's practice, became the heart of organisational development.

Nevertheless, many attempts to bring about change to organisations by strategies of organisational development have failed. Research has revealed that 45–75 per cent of change interventions in different types of organisations fail when compared to their initial goals (Fay & Lührmann, 2004). Leading experts on organisational change even estimate a failure rate of up to 90 per cent (Kotter & Cohen, 2002). The main reason for lack of success, or even fiascos, is that the organisation is not ready for change, and that means: there is no strong feeling of urgency spread over all parts of the organisation to change its own performance in order to survive in a changing environment (Kotter & Cohen, 2002).

If this is the case with enterprises and their employees, how much more it must apply to schools and their teachers. In many countries they suffer from a complete lack of competition and comparison, and consequently from an absence of a will to change, a lack of change competent management, and a lack of clear goals on where to change over to.

Why does change management fail?

Following Kotter and Cohen (2002), the most frequent reason for the failure of interventions in organisations is that it is not taken up by those whose behaviour is actually to be changed, be it staff members or be it the users of service organisations. This difficulty is about people and the feelings they associate with change: the disinclination to leave a comfortable situation, the insecurity that stems from replacing a safe well-mastered routine with a risky innovation, inferiority and mental overload that stems from the expectation of unforeseen obstacles that they cannot control, anxiety about failing and being responsible, resistance against change and against the expectation to live for others' ideas.

As Kotter & Cohen stated it: 'The central challenge in all eight stages [of change,] is changing people's behaviour. The central challenge is not strategy, not systems, not culture . . . Changing behaviour is less a matter of giving people analysis to influence their thoughts than helping them to see a truth to influence their feelings . . . The heart of change is in the emotions' (Kotter & Cohen, 2002: 2).

A core part of these emotions is about autonomy, empowerment, and control. Autonomy in the sense of basic human needs theory (Deci & Ryan, 2000) denotes the possibility to experience one's own self in any action that an individual undertakes; control is a slightly different concept that focuses on the possibility that the individual may control his or her environment by decision and action; consequently, empowerment can be seen as the characteristic of an organisation to offer open spaces and latitudes that allow an individual to set his or her own controls and experience autonomy (Dür, 2008).

If change management fails, because it does not appropriately relate to people in the sense of these concepts, then it seems that the 'Do!'-corner of the PDCA-cycle has a much too simplistic idea of what implementation at its core really is. Obviously, it is more than an imperative that can be adhered to or not; it is more and something different than the one-to-one-copy of a plan onto just another medium called 'reality'; it is even more than a translation of one communication into another, of one thought (in the leader's head) into another thought (in the co-worker's head). It seems to be a combination of changes in the medium and in the message. It is, therefore, better described as a metamorphosis like the change process that starts with a nymph and ends with a butterfly. A useful implementation theory must be able to describe and explain the process in between; in our case: between the nymph 'strategic decision of an organisation' and the butterfly 'individual behaviour'.

Organisation vs. the individual

The first two scientific theories of organisation were developed by a German sociologist and an American engineer: Max Weber's concept of bureaucracy, and the functionalist concept of the 'scientific organisation' by Frederic W. Taylor, known as Taylorism, are still of strong influence in the field. In both concepts, as different as they are, organisation was conceptualised as analogous to the structure of a machine, based on hierarchy, norms, sanctions and functionality (March & Simon, 1958). This machine model of organisation has continually informed theories of organisation as well as practices of management until the end of the twentieth century – and unfortunately still does (Adler, 1999; Daft & Marcic, 1998; Morgan, 1998). However, it became apparent that there is a blind spot in the machine model, and that is the person with his or her human complexity. For ethical and practical reasons, humans cannot be described and treated like machines, because they develop all sorts of reactance (March & Simon, 1958). As a consequence, an alternative concept of organisation was based on the model of an organism (Mayo, 1947). But the construction was still simplistic in seeing the organism as a living machine. This had an interesting consequence: the more individuals were seen as parts of this machine, the more their individuality and self-will became a problem and human organisation was about finding the right way to establish positive social relations. Modern management theories and concepts based on the organismic paradigm are hierarchy-sceptic, promoting human relations and aiming at a positive organisational culture. But they often only replace a mechanistic with a sociotechnical mode of thinking (Deeg & Weibler, 2008). They do so by treating the individual as an element of the organisation and thus blur the pathways of causal attribution of mistakes and failures: these then can be moved arbitrarily between managerial leadership and operative conduct. It is the big advantage of modern system theory to offer a theoretical framework that makes it possible to describe both organisations and individuals as distinct systems so that their relation can become a separate subject of investigation.

In the following we refer to the basic cybernetic theory of non-trivial machines from von Foerster (1984), to the biological theory of autopoiesis by Maturana and Varela (Varela, Maturana & Uribe, 1974), the logic of difference

(Spencer-Brown, 1969), the biological epistemology (Bateson, 1972) and to the application of these concepts in the specific system theory as presented by the German sociologist Niklas Luhmann (1995) (for English publications with reference to his organisation theory see Bakken & Tor, 2003; Nassehi, 2005; Seidl & Becker, 2006).

Basic epistemological and theoretical assumptions of system theory

Everything that exists is the result of its own fundamental operation that uses a particular distinction to make a difference between itself and its environment (Bateson, 1972; Luhmann, 2006; Spencer-Brown, 1969). To use Bateson's term: a system *is* 'a difference that makes a difference' (1972, 453). And to quote Spencer-Brown: 'Draw a distinction and a universe comes into being' (1969, v). This epistemological starting point breaks with the philosophical traditions of ontological and transcendental metaphysics and replaces such categorical logics[3] with a strict operational logic that puts the operation (of drawing a distinction) to the very beginning. Consequently, it operates to distinguish strictly between biological (somatic), mental and social systems, because these are obviously based on distinct operations, which are conceptualised as life, consciousness and communication (Luhmann, 1995; Seidl & Becker, 2006). These operations or systems, respectively, are not intertwined or conflated, but self-referential, meaning that each operation connects only to itself: only life produces life, only thoughts produce thoughts, only communication communicates – and consciousness, as Luhmann states with subtle humour, bothers itself about it (Luhmann, 1995).

Systems in that sense are conceptualised as autopoietic (self-reproducing) (Maturana & Varela, 1992; Varela, *et al.*, 1974), circular, historic, non-trivial machines (von Foerster, 1984), and that means that their output is not determined by the input from the environment, but relies on internal calculations (considerations) of the system itself. And this makes them unpredictable for an external observer. To describe non-trivial machines, von Foerster differentiates between two different functions (or competencies) that respond, one in a mechanistic way to the observed environment and the other to the self. The latter is the self-function of the system that only reproduces the self and maintains the autopoietic process. The point is that it is the self which influences and governs the functioning of all other functions. As an example, one could think of the (trivial) ability of a child to reproduce a poem after rehearsing it many times and of his or her inability to perform it when standing in front of an audience, because of an internal state of anxiety or feelings of shame and inferiority. It is obvious that more rehearsals would not solve this problem.

Although they are operationally closed, systems are open for observations in their environment. But they 'determine when, what and through which channels energy or matter is exchanged with the environment' (Seidl & Becker,

2006: 15). As for social and mental systems, the terms energy and matter must be replaced with sense. Operational closure and observational openness against the environment are the preconditions for the ability to adapt to other systems in a co-evolutionary process by internal arrangements.

Because observation (cognitive openness) is only possible from the backdrop of the internal state (operative closure) of the system, no information is imported from the environment into the system, but always self-produced by the system itself. 'The environment contains no information; the environment is as it is', as von Foerster states (1984: 263). Therefore, noise from the environment is only meaningful to the system if it can be related (i.e. if it makes a difference) to the operations of the system (Luhmann, 2003). This is to say that a system always combines self-reference and external reference and by that develops two options to attribute cognitions either to itself or to its environment. It is well-known, for example, that teachers feel responsible for positive learning effects of their students, but not for their errors and mistakes.

The most important consequence resulting from these theoretical constructions is that no system can operate within the boundary of another system. No one, for instance, can produce thoughts in another person's brain. And the thoughts of minds cannot be fully represented within communications, do not determine these and, therefore, also cannot navigate the way social systems take up and communicate about them. Since operations cannot cross the boundary of their system into another system, the concept of causality to describe the relation between systems is abandoned in system theory. There is circular causality within systems, but not causality nor interference or manipulation from outside. System theory therefore uses evolutionary theory and the concept of structural coupling (Weick, 1979) in order to explain why interactions between systems are possible without fully understanding the other system's complexity and how autonomous adaptations (variations and selections) on both sides lead to a dynamic homeostasis in their relations.

Function system, interaction and organisation

Social systems are defined by the operation of communication. Every communication and only communication is a social system, strictly differentiated from mental and organic or other biological and material systems.[4] Society then appears as the ensemble of all social systems, and it is meaningful to differentiate three types of social systems: function systems, interactions, and organisations (Nassehi, 2005; Seidl & Becker, 2006).

Function systems are defined as the big contexts of communications that are crystallising around societal functions like the production of laws (politics), jurisdiction (legal system), administration of scarcity (economy), production of knowledge (science), care for the sick (health care system), and so on. Function systems specify in a fundamental way what the system's output is and how it is achieved.

Interactions are defined as communication among present persons (Luhmann, 1995) and are fugitive and volatile, because they disappear as soon as one of the people leaves the situation. The peculiarity of interaction systems is this presence of bodies that are reciprocally interpreted as sign systems that inform about the mind. Interactions, therefore, especially when occurring in the context of organisations, add content to the communication, and since this content is about the personality, motives, emotions, sympathies and antipathies, it might be constructive in one kind of situation or gravely disturbing in another.

Organisations are characterised by their incomparably strong capacity of making decisions under the generalisable condition of uncertainty regarding the future and disagreement among those affected (Luhmann, 2003). In that sense, the autopoietic operation of organisations is making decisions, by which the purpose of the specific function system is organised. They are 'systems that consist of decisions and that by themselves produce the decisions of which they consist through the decisions of which they consist' (Seidl & Becker 2006: 28). Every decision, as soon as declared, becomes a premise for a next decision, either to do what the decision stipulates or to change the decision. The decision of a school, for example, to implement a certain health promotion programme is nothing less and nothing more than a frame for making new decisions in the course of its implementation. It provides descriptions (plans) of what somebody at some stage in the process has to decide to do. It is important to understand that the subsequent action is no longer an element of the social system organisation, but a product of the individual attributable to its structurally coupled mental and somatic system. The decision cannot absolutely determine the action.

This operative conception makes it possible to understand the different stages of implementation processes as a network of decisions on different levels of an organisation, and yet be permanently aware of the difference between communication and action, between the speech act or language game and the factual act or occupation related to the decision, between the willingness of an individual to comply and the ability to do so. In that sense, organisations and individuals are opposing each other and their relationship is basically confrontational. This is no recipe to keep them in a stable equilibrium of harmony, rather they both are well advised to learn to live with conflicting interests, and, as Luhmann (2003) suggests, learn to use the structured complexity that they represent for each other, for their own developments.

The school as an organisation

Decisions in schools are made typically on programmes like curricula, examination procedures, the schedule, and features of classroom management. These programmes define the so-called core process of a school. Compared with enterprises it is striking that schools mainly use conditional programmes, which have the format of an 'if–then' relation ('if this is the case, then do that'), and rarely use goal programmes (Seidl & Becker, 2006), that would allow for much more self-responsibility, creativity, and participation and self-control. This is because goal programmes predefine only the expected output, not the means to get there. Conditional programmes are very useful in some areas, for example, when it comes to safety systems in a nuclear power plant. Even in education they can be useful, when the aim is, for example, to automatise the mind–body coordination. But otherwise they are detrimental, if not destructive to creativity and innovation as well as to the experience of joy in one's work.

Furthermore, it is interesting to see that the dominance of conditional programmes holds true for teachers and students alike. Of course, students reflect teachers to be trivialising them and forcing them into a tight 'if–then' straightjacket. But teachers in turn also report themselves as being squeezed into the limitation of orders and commandments of superior structures from behind, and pupils' misbehaviour from the front.

The dominance of conditional programmes in schools is due to the limited degree of teachers' professionalism as compared, for example, with medical doctors. Since education changes the bodies, the thinking, feeling and behaving of children and by selection their social status as well, schools are so-called people processing and people changing organisations (Hasenfeld, 1983), in a similar way to hospitals. Professionalism is based on reliable, scientifically proven technologies and guarantees that the child will receive good education and the patient good medical care. While hospitals are true professional expert organisations in the sense of Mintzberg (1979), schools and teachers suffer from what Luhmann has called 'a technology deficit' (Luhmann, 2002). It is this technology deficit that teachers compensate with conditional programmes by which they trivialise their students (von Foerster, 1984): immobilisation, reduction of autonomy, intensification of dependency, neglecting of individual differences and collectivisation, standardisation of learning processes, and so on.

A further consequence of this technological deficit is the dominance of the interaction level in schools as opposed to the governance and leadership level (Luhmann, 2002). Since teachers can only partially rely on their technological qualifications, they tend to build their teaching on their own personal social and communication abilities. As a consequence, good teaching depends highly on the quality of the single teacher–student relationship, on the personal fit between teacher and pupil, on sympathies and antipathies, and on the social backgrounds of both.

Finally, because of the internal compartmentalisation of schools and the fact that teachers in secondary grades of most school systems are not exclusively attached to one particular class, it is pertinent that teachers neither develop a high degree of cohesion and cooperation with only a few colleagues nor a strong sense of responsibility for the performance of one specific or of any class. Encounters between teachers and classes, therefore, hardly condense to strong, confirming self-observations of the system. Instead, typecasting prejudices from teachers against classes and from classes against teachers go a long way and are even transferred over class and generation boundaries.

Modelling the organisation–individual relationship

From the backdrop of these descriptions of systems, organisations and schools, it becomes clear that interventions, be it from health promotion or any other quality oriented interest, are a far more complex and risky endeavour than the manuals on project management normally indicate. The generic model in Figure 3.1 delineates the stages of implementation that a health promotion programme must go through.

The model roughly differentiates four areas:

1.   the organisation;
2.   the individual;
3.   their social and material environments;
4.   the interaction between staff members (teachers) and users (students).

The organisation and the individual each consist of five boxes that represent the logical structure of Heinz von Foerster's non-trivial machine (von Foerster, 1984). The depiction of the interaction is more simplified, for interactions do not develop sustainable structures; they are represented by the three basic elements that constitute communication as a self-referent system (Luhmann, 1995). The environment is for the given purpose, not further specified. The plain arrows in the model signify circular-causal relations within a system; the dotted arrows signify the flow of information between systems, while the arrow points to the system, which is actively generating the information from its observations of the system where the arrow starts.

The five boxes of the organisation read as follows: (1) the organisation (based on a specific decision to observe) observes its specific environment and communicates the observation – in von Foerster's cybernetic model called input – internally as an irritation or a problem or a challenge in a very broad sense; this communication leads to either (4), an operative decision on how to handle this irritation, if strategic decisions for the actual case are available, or to (2), communications regarding possible strategic implications and necessary adaptations of the strategic set-up of the organisation; such strategic communications and considerations use and depend on (3), the given structures regarding staff and qualifications, communication channels (hierarchies), available resources in terms of time and money, valid policies on how to deal with this type of problem. Between (2) and (3) we find the basic self-referential process of the system: the organisation uses its structures, but might find that these are not useful and change or amend them. The goal of this stage is to adapt the system to the environmental challenge. This becomes the prerequisite for the preparation of the organisation's response, which is prepared by (4), the operative decisions in terms of making plans for reactions. The final step – originally called output – is (5), the communication of operative decisions and plans to those who have to re-orient their behaviour. While strategic decisions have the form of goals and

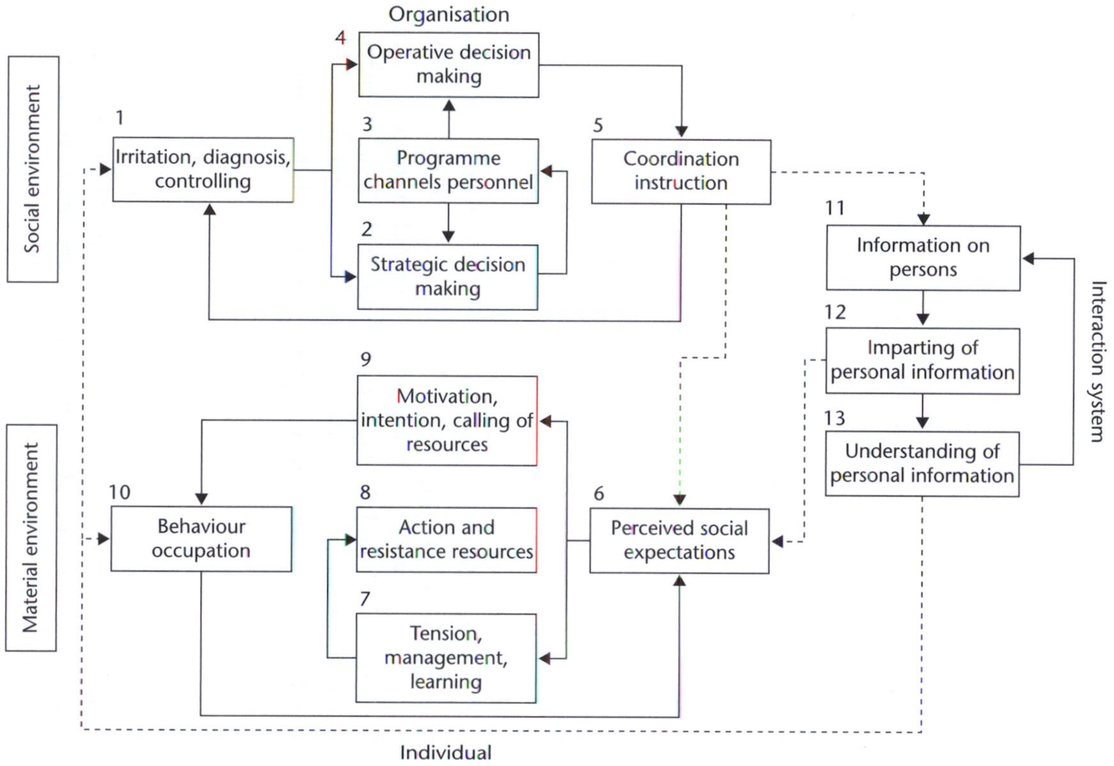
Organisation
Social environment
1
Irritation, diagnosis, controlling
4
Operative decision making
3
Programme channels personnel
2
Strategic decision making
5
Coordination instruction
11
Information on persons
12
Imparting of personal information
13
Understanding of personal information
Interaction system
Material environment
10
Behaviour occupation
9
Motivation, intention, calling of resources
8
Action and resistance resources
7
Tension, management, learning
6
Perceived social expectations
Individual

FIGURE 3.1 Model of the dynamic relations between the organisation, the individual and the interaction system

should-be states and while operative decisions have the form of plans and as-if conditions, the communication of plans must have the form of social expectations (imperatives) that at the same time are the template for all observations of real behaviour in (1) which decide upon whether the social expectations have been realised by the behaviour or disappointed. A second closure of the system is foreseen between (5) and (1), indicating that the whole procedure might move back and forth several times and that the system has got the ability to use own outputs as inputs and react to itself.

The model of the individual is likewise oriented on von Foerster's non-trivial machine. To translate the cybernetic abstractions for our purpose, the model uses distinctions and the terminology of Antonovsky's concept of salutogenesis (Antonovsky, 1987), which is also compatible with stress theory in terms of Selye (1977) and Lazarus (1991).

The model starts with box (6), perceptions of the individual, and since we are interested in his or her relation to the organisation, it is about perceptions concerning social expectations communicated in box (5). It is acknowledged that the body has its own perceptions, and that these are not necessarily mediated by mind processes, for example in the case of air pollution. But if behaviour change is to be triggered, then the body's perceptions must lead to mental perceptions. As with organisations, these perceptions may directly lead to (9), motives and intentions for immediate reactions, but will also unleash (7), arousals and tensions and therefore stimulate tension management. Tension management depends on (8), the mental structures, the personality, abilities like resilience or self-efficacy and competences in a broad sense called action and resistance resources by Antonovsky. Tension management and mental structures are mutually dependent: the potential of structures will improve to the same degree as tension management succeeds, which conversely depends on the potential of structures. This is why tension management could also be seen as a learning process. Dependent on the ability to manage tensions and on the competences that at a given moment are available and retrievable, the individual will develop (9), a behavioural intention, which is conceptualised as the intent 'I will . . .' combined with a concept of the action or occupation. In the cases of automatic behaviour (Bargh, 1994) the conscious 'I will . . .' might be obscured or even missing and only a concept of the action might be given, such as a habit or a routine. Since most things that people do in a day are driven by habits and routines, any behaviour change must attack the taken-for-grantednesses on which these are based and develop new behaviour/occupation concepts. This is the point where organisational change requires individual change in the sense of Scharmer (2007).

It is important to differentiate intensions and habits from (10), the factual behaviour that is observable for others outside the individual. It is this factual behaviour that the organisation (box 1) observes and that will lead to further communications and instigations. For this purpose, organisations use a very simple observation scheme, namely the difference of fulfilment and disappointment with regard to the initial plans and goals.

The role of the interaction system in the model is to facilitate the distinction between two types of communication, and communication contents that earlier have been described. This is the distinction between impersonal functional and personal contents. The personal and emotional sides of organisational matters are brought into play by individuals in interactions. The communication of plans and orders (box 5) might well be understood by the recipient (box 6), but not be accepted because of the tone in which instructions were given.

The long way of health promotion programmes from the adoption to changed behaviour

This generic model can be specified for intervention processes in organisations and make the whole process of implementation observable. When applied to school health promotion, the model reveals pitfalls as well as opportunities and might inspire implementation endeavours seen as the art of constructing meta-morphoses. For this purpose, the generic model is translated into the language of intervention, following the numbers of the boxes.

Box (1) *Programme selection*: An organisation defines a certain problem and decides to solve it with a health promotion programme. The question is: How to identify the right programme for this problem in that organisation? Schools normally do not have the capacity and the ability to conduct a diagnosis process that would set a reasonable frame for a selection procedure. Due to their partial blindness regarding their own processes and structures they would need a critical perspective from outside. National and international bodies and networks partially serve this need, but there is much room for improvement.

Box (2) *Project structures and Box (3)*

Box (3) *Programme adoption*: A strategic decision is necessary to put health promotion on the agenda and to support the chosen programme. A basic question is: do leaders claim ownership, assign resources etc.? There is a strong belief in school health promotion that nothing goes right at all, if the headteacher does not support the programme. With regard to the described dominance of the teacher–student interactions as opposed to leadership in schools, one is inclined to formulate the hypothesis that the principal's role is much overestimated. However, an increase of successes will depend on the establishment of stronger governance structures in schools. Even though the programme implementation is handed over to a teacher or a group of teachers, the responsibility and the line of reporting must be clear and obeyed. Otherwise the network of decisions will not be large nor strong enough for the high demands of the whole school approach.

Box (4) *Programme adaptation*: The programme becomes tailored to the conditions of the organisation. Plans for implementation are made. Questions are: How to adapt the programme? How to balance between necessary adaptation and fidelity? There are not so many highly standardised and evidence based school health promotion programmes. The majority are models with a high proportion of singular peculiarities that restrict generalisability. Therefore, they need to be applied to a specific school in a meaningful and reasonable manner, and this requires well-trained and skilled teachers. Furthermore, this requires time resources, which often are not available for teachers, or the assignment of time for health promotion is not clear. As a hypothesis one could assume that there is rather too little adaptation effort in schools and too much copy–paste fidelity – even towards programmes that do not warrant it. Teacher training should pick up on this issue to encourage understanding that adaptation is an important precondition in the implementation process, as long as it does not compromise the function of the original action suggested.

Box (5) *Commitment process*: The adapted programme and the implementation plans are communicated to staff and users: How to make the programme accepted in the school community? How can we promote it, who will take it on board? Commitment can diminish in the course of a project and must be constantly boosted. It has been reported that health promotion projects tend to meet with approval in children from middle class families and rather with disapproval in children from uneducated lower class families who, of course, may need it the most. The commitment process between teachers and students is burdened with all the unpleasant experiences and feelings that come with conditional programmes and trivialisation. To break through these limitations, smart health promotion programmes rely on authentic and sincere participation from the beginning.

Box (6) *Acceptance*: Single persons and groups have to accept the project and contribute to it. For each person the question will be: Shall I participate? Can I afford to participate? What is the benefit for me? Can I afford not to participate? As long as school health promotion does not promise to change basic difficulties of being a teacher and of being a student – and that means to really change core process features – it will be difficult to make it acceptable to those who suffer from these structures and processes the most. This is the point where negative emotions like anxiety or annoyance must be controlled and needs for autonomy, empowerment and control must be evoked.

Box (12) *Support*: The interactions with project leaders and others may strengthen or undermine the readiness to accept. Is the interaction climate supportive to successful negotiations? A positive climate cannot be ordered. It is easier to improve a good climate to a very good one than a bad climate to a less bad one. Nobody really knows what to do in such a situation, but one can assume that an intended behaviour change in some members of the organisation who are seen as role models and opinion leaders will be essential. Quality health promotion projects try to find these and organise face-to-face-communications.

Box (7) and (8) *Identification:* In order to overcome doubts and negative feelings, the individual needs to develop a high motivation and a sense of ownership. Will I be able to contribute substantially? Is this project 'my thing'? Collectivisation has been named as one typical school problem. If students treat health promotion like 'their thing', then the programme will need individualisation and diversification. Furthermore, if programmes have the same characteristics as normal school processes, then such identification is most unlikely.

Box (9) *Occupation concept:* The programme in the end consists of many single actions and tasks realized by specific persons. For that, they need occupation concepts that fit together with the initial plans. Questions are: How shall I do it? How can I make the plans come true? Occupational concepts are either transferred by role models or they need quite a time to be developed and tried out by the very person who is about to do it. The latter needs empowerment from the organisation in the sense of free spaces and the freedom to devote oneself to such inventions.

Box (10) *Behaviour/occupation performance:* The performance of any occupation is open to unforeseen disturbances from the environment and cannot absolutely be protected against them. The individual therefore will accommodate his or her behaviour with regard to such imponderables. Self–observation and self control can lead to Box (7), adjustments of the behaviour. Accommodation needs empowerment: the free space to experiment, adjust and re–adjust their own behaviour. Quality health promotion programmes do not present students and teachers with one more constraint in which to feel uncomfortable, but open spaces and areas where the tenets from the Ottawa Charter about self–determination and control over one's own living and working conditions can come true.

Box (11) The performed behaviour is observed by the organisation by means of evaluation. From evaluation, results produce new problems and irritations. Was the programme implemented successfully? Did the intended changes happen? Do the results of these changes meet expectations? If not, the cycle starts here again.

The implementation model for school health promotion presented above aims to capture and demonstrate the complexity of changing behaviours in individuals and organisations. Applying the system theory, the core questions that need to be addressed and answered to achieve change are identified. It is still left to the schools to develop motivation and capacity to deal with the required complexity of this Whole School Approach to change. Particular emphasis needs to be given to the individuals and their interactions if the process is to lead to real and sustainable change.

Notes

1   Acknowledgement to Benjamin Marent for proofreading and commenting.
2   PDCA (plan–do–check–act) is an iterative four-step management method used in business for the control and continuous improvement of processes and products. It is also known as the Deming circle/cycle/wheel, Shewhart cycle, control circle/cycle, or plan–do–study–act (PDSA); http: //en.wikipedia.org/wiki/PDCA, accessed 27th January 2012.
3   A categorical logic uses the difference of a subjective as opposed to an objective world as the epistemological precondition of cognition. This logic cannot handle the fact that the subjective is also part of the objective world.
4   In early debates on system theory in the 1980s, Luhmann once joked that, if social systems consisted of real human beings, then the hair-cutter would cut off pieces of society – and society would decrease when the hair-cutting business increased; and he found it a naïve and amusing idea to think that society consisted partly of communications, partly of feelings, partly of blood, and partly of oil, steel and rubber.

References

Adler, P. A. (1999). Building better bureaucracies. *Academy of Management Executive, 13*(4), 36–47.

Antonovsky, A. (1987). *Unraveling the Mystery of Health. How People Manage Stress and Stay Well.* San Francisco, CA: Jossey-Bass Inc.

Bakken, T. & Tor, H. (2003). *Autopoietic Organization Theory: Drawing on Niklas Luhmann's Social Systems Perspective.* Copenhagen: Copenhagen Business School Press.

Bargh, J. A. (1994). The Four Horsemen of automaticity: Awareness, efficiency, intention, and control in social cognition. In R. S. Wyer, Jr. & T. K. Srull (Eds), *Handbook of Social Cognition* (2nd edn, pp. 1–40). Hillsdale, NJ: Erlbaum.

Bateson, G. (1972). *Steps to an Ecology of Mind.* San Francisco, CA: Chandler.

Bricheno P., Brown S. & Lubansky, R. (2009). *Teacher Wellbeing: A Review of the Evidence.* London: Teacher Support Network.

Currie, C., Nic-Gabhainn, S., Godeau, E., Roberts, C., Smith, R., Currie, D., *et al.* (2008). *Inequalities in Young People's Health. HBSC International Report from the 2005/2006 Survey.* Copenhagen: WHO.

Daft, R. L. & Marcic, D. (1998). *Understanding Management.* Orlando, FL: Dreyden Press.

Deci, E. L. & Ryan, R. M. (2000). The "what" and "why" of goal pursuits: human needs and the self-determination of behavior. *Psychological Inquiry, 11*(4), 227–268.

Deeg, J. & Weibler, J. (2008). *Die Integration von Individuum und Organisation.* Wiesbaden: VS Verlag für Sozialwissenschaften.

Deming, W. E. (1986). *Out of the Crisis.* Cambridge, MA: MIT Center for Advanced Educational Studies.

Deschesnes, M., Martin, C. & Hill, A. J. (2003). Comprehensive approaches to school health promotion: how to achieve broader implementation? *Health Promotion International, 18*(4), 387–396.

Due, P. Lynch, J., Holstein, B. & Modvig, J. (2003): Socioeconomic health inequalities among a nationally representative sample of Danish adolescents. The role of different types of social relations. *Journal of Epidemiology and Community Health, 57*(9), S.692–698.

Dür, W. (2008). *Gesundheitsförderung in der Schule. Empowerment als systemtheoretisches Konzept und seine empirische Umsetzung.* Bern: Hans Huber.

Fay, D. & Lührmann, H. (2004). Current themes in organizational change. *European Journal of Work and Organizational Psychology, 13*, 113–119.

Flaschberger, E., Nitsch, M. & Waldherr, K. (2011). Implementing School Health Promotion in Austria: Experiences from a Pilot Training Course. *Health Promotion Practices, 13*(3), 364–369.

Hargreaves, L. G. (2008). The whole-school approach to eduation for sustainable development: From pilot projects to systemic change. *Policy & Practice: A Development Education Review, 6*, 69–74.

Hasenfeld, Y. (1983). *Human Service Organizations*. Englewood Cliffs, NJ: Prentice-Hall.

International Association for the Evaluation of Educational Achievement, (2008). International mathematics report: findings from IEA's trends in international mathematics and science study at the fourth and eighth grades. Retrieved from http://timssandpirls.bc.edu (accessed 21 September 2012).

Kotter, J. P. & Cohen, D. S. (2002). *The Heart of Change: Real Life Stories of How People Change Their Organizations*: Maidenhead: McGraw-Hill Professional.

Lazarus, R. S. (1991). *Emotion and Adaption*. London: Oxford University Press.

Luhmann, N. (1995). *Social Systems* (J. Bednarz, Jr. & D. Baecker, Trans.). Stanford, CA: Stanford University Press.

Luhmann, N. (2002). *Das Erziehungssystem der Gesellschaft*. Suhrkamp: Frankfurt am Main.

Luhmann, N. (2003) *Soziologie des Risikos*. Berlin/New York: De Gruyter.

Luhmann, N. (2006). System as difference organization: the critical journal on organization. *Theory and Society, 13*(1), 37–57.

March, J. M. & Simon, H. (1958). *Organizations*. New York: John Wiley & Sons.

Maturana, H. R. & Varela, F. J. (1992). *The Tree of Knowledge*. Boston, MA: Shambhala.

Mayo, E. (1947). *The Political Problem of Industrial Civilization. I. The modernization of a primitive community. II. Change and its social consequences. Two lectures delivered at a conference on human relations and administration, Harvard University, Graduate School of Business Administration, May 10 and 11, 1947*. Boston, MA: Division of Research, Graduate School of Business Administration, Harvard University.

Mintzberg, H. (1979). *The Structuring of Organizations*. New Jersey: Prentice-Hall.

Morgan, G. (1998). *Images of Organization: The Executive Edition*. San Francisco, CA: Berrett-Koehler.

Mukoma, W. & Flisher, A. J. (2004). Evaluations of health promoting schools: a review of nine studies. *Health Promotion International, 19*(3), 357–368.

Nassehi, A. (2005). Organizations as decision machines. Niklas Luhmann's theory of organized social systems. In J. Campbell & R. Munro (Eds), *Contemporary Organization Theory*. Oxford: Blackwell.

OECD (2010a). *Improving Health and Social Cohesion through Education*. Retrieved from http://www.oecd.org.

OECD (2010b). *PISA 2009 Results: Overcoming Social Background – Equity in Learning Opportunities and Outcomes (Volume II)*. Retrieved from http: //www.oecd.org.

OECD (2010c). *PISA 2009 Results: What Students Know and Can Do – Student Performance in Reading, Mathematics and Science (Volume I)*. Retrieved from http://www.oecd.org.

Rasmussen, M., Mogens, T. D., Holstein, B. E., Poulsen, L. H. & Due, P. (2005). School connectedness and daily smoking among boys and girls: the influence of parental smoking norms. *European Journal of Public Health, 15*(6), 607–612.

Ravens-Sieberer, U., Freeman, J., Kokonyei, G., Thomas, C. A. & Erhart, M. (2009).

School as a determinant for health outcomes – a structural equation model analysis. *Health Education, 109*(4), 342–356.

Samdal, O., Wold, B., Klepp, K. I. & Kannas, L. (2000). Students' perception of school and their smoking and alcohol use: a cross-national study. *Addiction Research, 8*(2), 141–167.

Scharmer, O. C. (2007). *Theory U: Leading from the Future as it Emerges.* Cambridge, MA: The Society for Organizational Learning.

Seidl, D. & Becker, K. H. (2006). Organizations as distinction generating and processing systems: Niklas Luhmann's contribution to organization studies. *The Critical Journal on Organization, Theory and Society, 13*(1), 9–35.

Selye, H. (1977). *Stress. Lebensregeln vom Entdecker des Stress-Syndroms.* Reinbek bei Hamburg: Rowohlt.

Spencer-Brown, G. (1969). *Laws of Form.* London: Allen and Unwin.

St Leger, L., Young, I., Blanchard, C. & Perry, M. (2010). *Promoting Health in Schools. From evidence to action.* Saint Denis Cedex: IUHPE.

Stewart-Brown, S. (2006). What is the evidence on school health promotion in improving health or preventing disease and, specifically, what is the effectiveness of the health promoting schools approach? *Health Evidence Network Report.* Copenhagen: WHO Regional Office for Europe.

Torsheim, T. & Wold, B. (2001). School-related stress, school support and somatic complaints: A general population study. *Journal of Adolscent Research, 16*(3), 293–303.

Varela, F. J., Maturana, H. R. & Uribe, R. B. (1974). Autopoiesis: The organization of living system, its characterization and a model. *BioSystems, 5*(4), 187–196.

von Foerster, H. (1984). *Observing Systems (The Systems Inquiry Series).* Seaside, CA: Intersystems Publications.

Weick, K. E. (1979). *The Social Psychology of Organizing.* Reading, MA: Addinson-Wesley.

World Health Organization (WHO), (1986). Ottawa Charter for Health Promotion. *Health Promotion International, 1*(4), iii–v.

4

THEORY BASED COMPONENTS FOR IMPLEMENTATION OF HEALTH PROMOTING SCHOOLS[1]

Oddrun Samdal and Louise Rowling

Implementation of health promoting schools is not a straightforward implementation of a pre-package programme, which in itself is fairly complex (Durlak, 2003). As demonstrated in Chapters 2 and 3 the implementation of health promoting schools needs to address individual change through organisational change. Denman (1999: 216) highlighted that 'Health promoting schools approach to practice requires the management and organisational structures to be supportive and for policies to be in place which are coherent, comprehensive and reached by consensus'. Health promoting schools may thus be seen as an approach or framework for action that parallels implementation of a policy or diffusion approach, which prior to the implementation process requires operationalisation of actions to meet policy and framework aims (Guldbrandsson & Bremberg, 2006; Rogers, 2003).

Labelling health promoting schools as a policy approach is particularly relevant as it was initiated by three major policy bodies in Europe: the European Commission, the European Parliament and World Health Organization, aiming at influencing national educational and health policies for promoting health in and through school (Burgher, Rasmussen & Rivett, 1999). Previous research has suggested that the adoption and implementation of health promotion packages and programmes in general (Durlak & DuPre, 2008) and public health policy, in particular in the school setting, are underdeveloped and under-researched (Holthe, Larsen & Samdal, 2011). Therefore, more research is required to understand the processes by which a policy initiative such as the health promoting school needs to be adapted and implemented in schools to meet its objectives (McGraw *et al.*, 2000).

At the launch of the European Network of Health Promoting Schools the following aim was formulated: 'The Health Promoting School aims at achieving healthy lifestyles for the whole school population by developing supportive environments conducive to the promotion of health' (Burgher, Rasmussen & Rivett, 1999). The whole school population thus includes both students and staff. In addition, the means to achieve the aim was identified: 'A Health Promoting School uses its *management structures*, its internal and external *relationships*, its *teaching and learning styles* and its methods of establishing synergy with its *social environment* to create the means for pupils, teachers and all those involved in everyday school life to take control over and improve their physical and emotional health.'

To meet the objectives of a health promoting school, an organisational change process is required as the actions wanted include a continuous process of improving school activities and relationships within the organisation to promote the health and well-being of all stakeholders at school. To accommodate organisational change in school, researchers have identified implementation strategies with varying foci and levels of specificity. Hargreaves and colleagues (2001) have through systematic and comprehensive studies with teachers and school leaders identified five factors important for development of organisational change processes in school:

1.   school leadership;
2.   school structures;
3.   teacher culture;
4.   professional learning;
5.   professional discretion.

With a similar aim, Daft (1999) has identified three core strategies for implementation of change processes in a school setting:

1.   providing direction in line with overall school aims and visions;
2.   aligning teacher and school efforts to achieve commitment towards an intervention;
3.   enabling the school to conduct the needed actions through resource and time allocation, and professional development.

A parallel approach to organisational change is taken through the concept of building organisational capacity (Elias, Zins, Graczyk & Weissberg, 2003; Flaspohler, Duffy, Wandersman, Stillman & Maras, 2008; Harris & Lambert, 2003; Hopkins & Jackson, 2003; Larsen & Samdal, 2007; Mihalic, Irwin, Fagan, Ballard & Eliott, 2004). Hopkins and Jackson (2003) have suggested that organisational capacity is composed of four components: (1) contribution, (2) alignment, (3) support, and (4) shared values.

Although slightly different in numbers and content, the three sets of strategies identify the same or similar categories of themes and components. The role of the school leadership seems to be one such category. This is explicitly identified by Hargreaves and colleagues (2001) and implicitly addressed by Daft (1999) through his concept of providing direction, which is a key feature of the leadership role. Likewise, although less evident, all the components identified by Hopkins & Jackson (2003) require strong leadership to be successful. Identification of the key function of the school leadership is further supported by educational research and research on health promoting schools in establishing successful school change (Deschesnes, Couturier, Laberge & Campeau, 2010; Fullan, 2008; McBride, Midford & Cameron, 1999).

A second cross cutting category, as mentioned in Chapter 2, is the concept of establishing readiness for change; i.e. to prepare an organisation and the participants for their participation in implementing actions to achieve aims of change (Elias *et al.*, 2003; Weiner *et al.*, 2009). This concept is explicitly highlighted in the second strategy, alignment, in the listing by both Daft (1999) and Hopkins and Jackson (2003). Alignment processes aim at providing direction so that the participants move in the same direction. This requires that they share the beliefs and values of the implementation aims and processes and are willing to work collaboratively to achieve the aims of change (Fullan & Huberman, 1992). Thus, Hopkins and Jackson's fourth component, shared values, further highlights the core aim of building readiness through alignment processes. Similarly, their component of 'contribution' may also stimulate readiness and motivation. In this regard, it is important that the school executives provide leadership and allow teachers to contribute to the change process and also share contradicting beliefs, knowledge, and attitudes, but still aiming for developing a set of shared values among the staff. This dialogue approach may seem to meet the requirement for communication and interaction between the participants as highlighted in system theory in Chapter 3. The alignment process is thus an important part of achieving active participation and shared values among the staff. Looking at Hargreaves and colleagues' (2001) components numbers 3–5 – teacher culture, professional learning, and professional discretion – they also address issues of alignment and shared values. The alignment process is more precisely about addressing the teacher culture and teachers' professional discretion by taking account of the teachers' views, practices and competencies and not forcing a change process that will not be accepted by the teachers. Allowing time to anchor the change process within the school culture and the school's aims and visions is important to achieve successful change. The importance for a successful change process to meet a school's overall goals and activities has also be identified in other educational changes studies (Elias *et al.*, 2003; Larsen & Samdal, 2007; Viig & Wold, 2005).

A final cross cutting category of the three presented implementation strategies for achieving change in school is related to organisational facilitation of the change process in terms of both an individual focus on teachers and the provision of the conditions to enable changed practice. This is covered in Daft's third strategy highlighting the importance of resource and time allocation and teacher training. Resource and time allocation can be seen to parallel Hargreaves and colleagues' component of school structure, whereas their component of professional learning may tap Daft's focus on teacher training. Similarly Hopkins and Jackson's (2003) support component addresses the importance of both structural and emotional support to achieve change. Previous research also highlights that the allocation of resources and time contributes to facilitate change and that lack thereof can be detrimental to a successful change process (Fullan & Huberman, 1992; Mihalic *et al.*, 2004). Thus, prior to the initiation of a change process it is crucial that needs for money, time, materials, and personnel are assessed and adequately ensured as a prerequisite for the change process. Further, professional development is needed to develop the knowledge and skills so that the staff can contribute to successful change through their practices (Mihalic *et al.*, 2004). Moreover, the professional development may also be seen to parallel Hargreaves and colleagues' component of professional learning. The professional development will moreover promote motivation and collective ownership of the implementation process (Fullan & Huberman, 1992), factors important for teachers' willingness to use their capacity and time in the on-going change process. Other than resources, time and professional development, practices like participation and support (Viig & Wold, 2005), and overall implementation climate (Weiner *et al.*, 2008), have also been identified as core elements of successful implementation.

Further, Harris and Lambert (2003) have observed that schools having the capacity to implement change are also more likely to sustain any improvement over time. In order to stimulate research based practice, demonstrated to be successful for implementation of change processes specifically aiming at promoting health in school, it is vital to identify factors for this more specified aim of change. The rest of the chapter is therefore allocated to this aim and builds on two papers recently published by the authors, where one paper aimed at identifying the components and highlighting their theoretical rationale (Samdal & Rowling, 2011) and the other addressed the practical implications of the identified components (Rowling & Samdal, 2011).

Building on the above theoretical framework and aim, a meta-analysis was conducted to identify core implementation components for achieving the aims of health promoting schools. Full description of the methodology is detailed in Samdal & Rowling (2011). Eight sources were identified (Aldinger *et al.*, 2008; Bond, Glover, Godfrey, Butler & Patton, 2001; Deschesnes, Martin & Hill, 2003; Felner *et al.*, 2001; Hoyle, Samek & Valois, 2008; Inchley, Muldoon & Currie, 2007; McBride, 2000; McBride *et al.*, 1999; Samdal, Viig & Wold, 2010) and from these eight components were extracted:

1. preparing and planning for school development;
2. policy and institutional anchoring;
3. professional development and learning;
4. leadership and management practices;
5. relational and organisational support context;
6. student participation;

7. partnership and networking;
8. sustainability.

Table 4.1 lists the sources and the components extracted from each of them. Below, the theoretical foundations will be elaborated on for each of the components to underscore the component's relevance for implementation of health promoting schools. A summary table (Table 4.2) of the components and their theoretical foundation is provided at the end.

Preparing and planning for school development

More than half of the sources identified the need to prepare the school for implementing the health promoting school approach (Bond *et al.*, 2001; Deschesnes *et al.*, 2003; Inchley *et al.*, 2007; McBride *et al.*, 1999; Samdal *et al.*, 2010). Some of them highlighted the usefulness of applying programme theory or programme planning models such as Green and Kreuter's (2005) PRECEDE model, to help identify which theoretical constructs should be addressed in the intervention when aiming to achieve organisational and individual level change. The programme planning models give attention to 'starting out' by identifying a clear aim for the change process, then performing a data collection and analysis of the current situation aiming to identify strengths and activities to build on and gaps and need for change. Further, the planning models frequently differentiate between individual and organisational components. They highlight that knowledge, skills and motivation are important individual components for participation in change processes, and that resource management and physical and structural components are important organisational components to facilitate the change process.

The planning models also emphasise the importance of planning the total implementation phase by building on implementation theory on how to implement actions, to achieve the aim of the intervention most successfully (Weiner, Lewis & Linnan, 2009). In this initial planning phase it is vital to identify concrete policies, structures and practices for the total implementation phase to anchor the health promoting school policy approach in the school organisation. The planning phase constitutes a core element of alignment processes that can stimulate readiness and commitment for change among all relevant stakeholders. This was identified in the introduction of the chapter to be crucial for a successful implementation process (Elias *et al.*, 2003; Flaspohler *et al.*, 2008; Sabatier, 1997; Stith *et al.*, 2006; Weiner *et al.*, 2009). Weiner and colleagues (2009) draw on Bandura's (1998) notions of goal commitment and collective efficacy when they explain the readiness concept. Goal commitment and collective efficacy is about stimulating shared values and beliefs that a proposed initiative is of importance for the organisation. The underlying principle of building readiness for a health promoting school policy approach is thus to establish beliefs that health promoting changes in the organisational climate of the school will also contribute to

TABLE 4.1 Overview of sources and the implementation components for implementation of health promoting schools

Source	Focus of article	Theoretical/ Conceptual base	Terminology of components used in the sources	Proposed common terminology for implementation components
Aldinger et al., 2008 Keywords: Health Promoting Schools, school health, China	A report of national implementation of health promoting schools (scaling up previous pilot phase)	Health promoting schools Implementation theory	a. Pre-implementation (entry point, committee, work plan) b. Implementation (mobilisation, prioritising, popularising, community participation, role modelling, training, new teaching and learning methods c. Monitoring and evaluation (process and outcome, holistic approach)	1) Preparing and planning 2) Policy and institutional anchoring 3) Professional development and learning* 4) Leadership and management 6) Student participation 7) Partnerships and networking* 8) Sustainability
Bond et al., 2001 Keywords: School change, school environments, capacity building, health promotion, student engagement, student well-being, Gatehouse Project	Empirical report on Australian programme to promote student engagement and school connectedness as the way to improve emotional well-being and learning outcomes.	Health promoting schools System change through capacity building	a. School-based adolescent health team b. Student surveys to identify risk and protective factors in each school c. Identification and implementation of effective strategies in project management d. External consultant/critical friend	1) Preparing and planning 2) Policy and institutional anchoring 3) Professional development and learning* 4) Leadership and management 5) Relational and organisational support context 7) Partnerships and networking*

Deschesnes, *et al.*, 2003 *Keywords*: Critical issues, comprehensive approaches, literature review, school health promotion	Literature review of comprehensive school health promotion/ health promoting schools		a. Negotiated planning and coordination to support the comprehensive, integrated nature of the approach b. Intersectoral action to actualise the partnership between school, family and community c. Political and financial support from policy makers d. Evaluative research as a support to implementation	1) Preparing and planning★ 2) Policy and institutional anchoring 5) Relational and organisational support context 7) Partnerships and networking
Felner *et al.*, 2001 *Keywords*: STEP, HiPlaces, prevention, restructuring, whole school improvement	Empirical report of health promoting schools in Colorado school district, USA	Eco-developmental school improvement theory based research model	a. Structural/organisational characteristics b. Attitudes, norms and beliefs of staff c. Climate/empowerment/experiential characteristics d. Capacity/skills e. Practice/procedural variables	1) Preparing and planning★ 3) Professional development and learning★ 5) Relational and organisational support context
Hoyle *et al.*, 2008 *Keywords*: Health promoting schools, capacity building, continuous improvement, school health, school improvement	Empirical report on two North-American projects based on building principles of prevention and promotion into whole school change	Organisational capacity building in schools and districts	a. Visionary/effective leadership and management structures (including coordinator) b. Extensive internal and external supports (structured approaches) c. Development and allocation of adequate resources (fiscal and human) d. Supportive policies and procedures e. On-going, embedded professional development	1) Preparing and planning 2) Policy and institutional anchoring 3) Professional development 4) Leadership and management 5) Relational and organisational support context 7) Partnerships and networking 8) Sustainability

(Continued)

TABLE 4.1 (*Continued*)

Source	Focus of article	Theoretical/ Conceptual base	Terminology of components used in the sources	Proposed common terminology for implementation components
Inchley et al., 2007 *Keywords*: Health promoting schools, process evaluation, implementation	Evaluation report on health promoting schools projects in Scotland	Processes involved in developing and implementing health promoting schools	a. School ownership and empowerment b. Leadership and management c. Collaboration d. Integration of new into existing practices	1) Preparing and planning 2) Policy and institutional anchoring 4) Leadership and management★ 5) Relational and organisational support context 6) Student participation 7) Partnerships and networking 8) Sustainability
McBride et al., 1999; McBride, 2000 *Keywords*: School, health promotion framework	Empirical report on development of an Australian model for health promoting schools implementation	Systems theory of organisational change	a. Process (needs assessment, school community, school management, school health promotion contributing to comprehensive school health promotion) b. Critical individuals (gateway personnel, key decision makers and workers) c. Supports and strategies (management factors and health promotion factors) d. Evaluation	1) Preparation and planning 3) Professional development and learning 4) Leadership and management 5) Relational and organisational support context 7) Partnerships and networking

Samdal et al., 2010 Keywords: Health promoting schools, implementation, systematic approach, sustainability	Empirical report of implementation of health promoting schools in Norway	Planning and implementation model for health promotion	a. Goal clarity b. No goal conflict c. Adequate change d. Familiar methodology e. Complexity f. Motivation and personal interest g. The role of management h. Integration of the project in the school policy i. Implementation strategy (top down/bottom up) j. Time and economy	1) Preparing and planning 2) Policy and institutional anchoring 4) Leadership and management* 5) Relational and organisational support context 6) Student participation 7) Partnerships and networking

*Only one of the two aspects included in this component was covered by this source.

Source: Samdal and Rowling, 2011, © Emerald Publishing Group, reprinted with permission.

students' development and learning as this is the overall goal of education. When stakeholders are aligned, motivated and ready for the implementation process they are also more likely to spend time and energy on agreed actions. This increases the likelihood that the actions will be implemented with fidelity and thereby have the intended impact.

As part of the planning approach several of the sources identified in the meta-analysis highlighted the usefulness of establishing a coordination team both for the development of the actions needed to become a health promoting school and for the implementation approach (Hoyle *et al.*, 2008; McBride *et al.*, 1999; Samdal *et al.*, 2010). Such a team would, in collaboration with stakeholders, have to identify topics/areas to meet local needs and develop actions to initiate and guide the organisational change process. In line with organisational change theory, the coordination team would have to work closely with the leadership of the school as the leadership has the key role of anchoring and facilitating the change process (Heward, Hutchins & Keleher, 2007; Hopkins & Jackson, 2003). Some of the sources suggested that the leadership be part of or even spearhead the coordination team. The aim is to ensure that the leadership is committed and positive to both the implementation of the health promoting school policy, and the actions needed to meet the policy aims (Inchley *et al.*, 2007; Samdal *et al.*, 2010).

The seven other implementation components presented below should typically be addressed in the planning phase to prepare for the implementation of the health promoting school policy. Further, these components should also specifically constitute agenda points for the coordination committee in terms of what they need to emphasise throughout the implementation process.

Policy and institutional anchoring

Three of the sources from the meta-analysis on implementation components for health promoting schools identify inclusion of the aims and activities in the school's policy plan (Bond *et al.*, 2001; Hoyle *et al.*, 2008; Samdal *et al.*, 2010). Indirectly, several of the other sources also address the importance of institutional anchoring through establishment of routines (Felner *et al.*, 2001), or development of ownership and resource allocation (Deschesnes *et al.*, 2003; McBride *et al.*, 1999). A written policy helps to ensure that priority will be given from the leadership through allocation of resources to the actions suggested. Further, the policy document is intended to commit all stakeholders to work towards achieving the agreed aims. An important element of the policy document is how it has been developed and agreed. A good policy development process spearheaded by the leadership would involve anchoring among, and involvement of all relevant stakeholders. In this way the stakeholders have had a say and an opportunity to influence the aims and objectives, and hopefully are more likely to be aligned and motivated to meet the agreed objectives. An objective in the policy document thus reflects and reinforces a decision taken through a consultative process by school leadership and stakeholders. A strong institutional anchoring is built on a combination of top-down initiatives from the leadership and bottom-up inputs and developments from the stakeholders. This makes achieving the objectives more realistic, as it is based on the school's competence and resources and the stakeholders' motivation to contribute (Heward et al., 2007; Hopkins & Jackson, 2003).

Professional development and learning

In accordance with Hargreaves and colleagues observation: 'Complex changes cannot be achieved without considerable learning' (Hargreaves et al., 2001: 169), the majority of the sources emphasise the importance of professional development and learning for successful implementation and change (Bond et al., 2001; Felner et al., 2001; Hoyle et al., 2008; Mihalic et al., 2004; Samdal et al., 2010). Professional development is meant all courses and learning opportunities that are organised outside the school premises. Frequently the content is decided by local school authorities and addresses knowledge more than skill development. Professional learning, on the other hand takes place at the school premises and is based on what the school needs or wants (a bottom-up approach) (Darling-Hammond, 2009; Fullan, Cuttress & Kilcher, 2009). The content is a mixture of knowledge, attitudes, skills, aspirations and behaviour depending on what the school and its stakeholders find is needed (Easton, 2008). The relevance of professional development and learning is evident in that the teachers are the core change agents in school-based change processes. Their competence and understanding of what to achieve by the health promoting school policy approach and how to achieve the agreed objective is therefore vital to the success and impact of the implementation of the health promoting organisational change process. Only when teachers know and feel competent in what to do can they contribute to achieve change. Professional development and learning can also be considered to be part of a teacher's everyday life in that they are invited and expected to participate in ongoing discussions on how to initiate and support school development and change. Openness to change is found to be a prerequisite for choosing to take part in change action (Fullan, 2001) and openness is likely to be stimulated by perceived competence and professional development.

Professional development and learning establish a critical base for building organisational capacity for change (Flaspohler et al., 2008; Hopkins & Jackson, 2003). Such capacity is found to be central for developing the necessary understanding, motivation and skills for the change process needed in the implementation of the health promoting school policy, as also advocated by some of the sources (Bond et al., 2001; Hoyle et al., 2008).

Leadership and management practices

The leadership is frequently considered the gatekeeper for change (Fullan, 2001) and thereby recognised as a core agent for stimulating and leading change processes in school (Hallinger, 2003; Hattie, 2009; Larsen & Samdal, 2008; Samdal, 2008; Senge, 2006). The key role of the school executive is also identified by the majority of the sources addressing successful implementation of school health promotion (Aldinger *et al.*, 2008; Hoyle *et al.*, 2008; Inchley *et al.*, 2007; McBride *et al.*, 1999; Samdal *et al.*, 2010). The role of the school leader is recognised as important for developmental work in schools.

Understanding and performance of leadership varies across countries due to political, economic and educational circumstances (Thomas, Parsons & Stears, 1998). Sometimes the concept primarily addresses the management of human and financial tasks, while ignoring the processes of leadership in terms of providing vision and goals for the organisation. A balance of leadership and management is, however, needed to achieve successful organisational development and change (Donaldson, 2001; Farrell, Meyer, Kung & Sullivan, 2001; Kam, Greenberg & Walls, 2003; Neil, McEwen, Carlisle & Knipe, 2001).

When in the leadership role the primary function is to develop and nurture readiness and motivation for change; in this process the leadership needs to balance external requirements and perceived internal capacity. Fullan (2001) has identified the complexity of the leadership role when he shows that a great mixture and variation of competencies are needed: having a clear vision and moral purpose; understanding change processes; having the capacity to build relationships and knowledge and ensure group coherence. In particular, the development and stimulation of professional learning through focusing on visions, competence building and motivational strategies is found to be a key function in the leadership role as this constitutes the basis for all development and change (Fullan, 2001). In their visionary and motivational roles leaders also represent an important role model for the stakeholders in terms of values and behaviours that are wanted and expected with regard to the change process they are undergoing (Bandura, 1998). Further, asking stakeholders how they are performing changes in their practice, and how they experience them, will also stimulate reflections and motivate for continued contribution.

Management is the other key part of the leadership role. In this role, focus is on ensuring structures and resources that stimulate the needed change practices (Leithwood *et al.*, 2007). Examples of such facilitation are resource allocation for professional development and teaching schedules allowing for teacher collaboration and exchange of experiences.

Relational and organisational support context

The majority of the sources identifying components for successful implementation of health promotion policy in schools, advocate the importance of organisational and contextual/relational support for implementing health promoting schools. This is also supported by implementation theory as a critical component, primarily operationalised as climate and culture (Boyd, 2006; Hargreaves *et al.*, 2001), or organisational capacity (Flaspohler *et al.*, 2008; Hopkins & Jackson,

2003). It further involves development of structures, strategies and practices which facilitate smooth and efficient implementation of actions and activities (Weiner *et al.*, 2009). The climate and culture provides relational support (Bandura, 1998) whereas organisational structures, including timetabling, physical environment and fiscal resources, constitute organisational support (Leithwood *et al.*, 2007).

In many ways the component of relational and organisational support context merges and includes all the other seven components for the needed change process in implementation of health promoting schools. Therefore it is vital that the coordinating committee works closely with the leadership in identifying actions and structures to support the development of a stimulating relational and organisational support context. As outlined above, the leadership in their management role are in control of both the resources and structures (organisational support). Additionally, in their leadership role they are responsible for stimulating alignment and motivation for achieving the health promoting school policy objectives (Bond *et al.*, 2001; Elias *et al.*, 2003; Sabatier, 1997). Of specific importance in this regard may be to organise more systematic opportunities for teachers to share and discuss their experiences. Research demonstrates the effectiveness of such discussion on the motivation for contribution and the success of the organisational change process (Kallestad & Olweus, 2003). The support context constituted by such discussion groups may be seen to build on social learning theory (Bandura, 1998) where stimulating a good climate for sharing experiences provides role models for successful behaviours, as well as opportunities for receiving social support to tackle challenges in difficult change processes.

The importance of students connecting to schools through a positive environment is also established, showing its importance both for students' life satisfaction and for their academic achievement (Danielsen, Samdal, Hetland & Wold, 2009; Samdal, Wold & Bronis, 1999; Samdal, Nutbeam, Wold & Kannas, 1998). Young people who cope successfully at school seem to draw on the support of teachers and peers in the school environment. Perhaps these adolescents develop positive coping responses through experiencing acceptance from peers, appropriate warmth and supervision from their teachers and through having safe opportunities to demonstrate competence in their school environments.

Student participation

Only one of the eight sources identifying components for implementation of health promoting schools (Inchley *et al.*, 2007) suggested student participation as an explicit implementation component, although Aldinger and colleagues (2008) and Samdal and colleagues (2010) mentioned the importance of involving the students. Due to its inclusion and perceived importance from the establishment of the health promoting school approach (Barnekow *et al.*, 2006; Buijs, 2009; Jensen & Simovska, 2005; Parsons, Stears & Thomas, 1996), it is included in the list of core implementation components for health promoting schools. Student participation involves the target group and thereby also meets one of the core principles of health promotion.

Building on relational pedagogy, student participation may be considered both a means and a goal to achieve motivation for health and learning (Boyd, MacNeill & Sullivan, 2006). Making decisions, being heard and also having the skills to see a task through and do it well, is found to result in a greater sense of control; doing something that has a bigger purpose and that students can 'believe in' gives them meaning; and working with others and being part of something bigger enhances connectedness (Wieranga *et al.* 2002). This reasoning is also in line with self-determination theory which postulates that satisfaction of three basic needs: autonomy, relatedness and competences, stimulates intrinsic motivation which again is basis for general well-being (Deci & Ryan, 2000). This implies that students who experience that their contributions are sought and valued are likely to be more intrinsically motivated for school and this may then positively influence both their academic achievement and overall well-being (Danielsen *et al.*, 2009).

Conversely, it has been observed that students in low-autonomy supported environments learn less effectively and report lower motivation (Deci & Ryan, 2000; Reeve & Jang, 2006). From this it can be hypothesised that students who have been given the opportunity for self regulation, that involves shared decision making with peers and adults, are more likely to develop intrinsic motivation and experience higher motivation for learning and higher levels of school and life satisfaction than students who are not given such opportunities. According to Larson (2000) intrinsic motivation in combination with concerted action over time will result in development of initiative, which is seen as an important competence for current and adult civic engagement. Larson (2000) believes that school by nature is not a setting where students are likely to develop initiative, but according to his reasoning, if these conditions could be created, school may still have the potential to develop student initiative. Schools where students, as part of daily practice, are allowed to initiate and influence decisions and actions, provide the context for the core elements of initiative development to come together. In line with health promotion this provides students with empowering conditions. Research has also demonstrated that students feel empowered when asked for their opinion and have developed skills to listen to others' arguments, and their empowerment helps them to achieve learning goals and develop self-reliance in their thinking (Stefanou *et al.*, 2004). Following the principles of Larson (2000) student participation may contribute to development of skills important for current and future civic engagement (Jensen and Simovska, 2005) that will nurture healthy working lives and strong democracies.

Partnership and networking

Half of the sources addressing implementation components for health promoting schools identified the importance for schools to establish partnerships and networking as part of their endeavour to become a health promoting school (Aldinger *et al.*, 2008; Deschesnes *et al.*, 2003; Inchley *et al.*, 2007; Samdal *et al.*, 2010). The same sources also highlighted the challenges the schools are likely to meet in this process. As a starting point, schools tend to look upon partners from a self-centred point of view, either as funding sources or someone who could help the schools to meet their aims. However, only when partnerships and networking are mutually supportive are they found to contribute to the successful health promoting school development (Boot, van Assama, Hesdal & de Vries, 2010; Deschesnes, Couturier *et al.*, 2010; Deschesnes *et al.*, 2003; Deschesnes, Trudeau & Kébé, 2010; Inchley *et al.*, 2007; Leurs *et al.*, 2005; Tjomsland, Larsen, Samdal & Wold, 2010; Viig, Tjomsland & Wold, 2010).

In a mutual partnership it is reasonable to assume that intersectoral collaboration between health and education ensures efficient use of resources and competence (Allensworth, Wyche, Lawson & Nicholson, 1995). In the health promoting schools approach the health sector would be expected to have the technical knowledge about the principles of health promotion, whereas the education sector is knowledgeable on how these principles can be applied and implemented in an educational setting. In order for a partnership to be functional it is also vital to emphasise shared vision and decision making to stimulate a mutual learning process (Deschesnes *et al.*, 2003; Deschesnes, Couturier *et al.*, 2010) stimulating development of organisational capacity for both or all partners (Flaspohler *et al.*, 2008; Hopkins & Jackson, 2003). By sharing experiences as well as tasks and responsibilities, it is also likely that a shared commitment towards common goals will be established, and thereby increase the likelihood of giving priority towards achieving them.

The school is a setting of high interest for the health sector to cooperate with, given its strong potential of promoting health from childhood and also to reach the parent population. For a functional partnership it is important that the health sector understands the key aims of education and how health promotion can contribute to these. This is of particular relevance as previous studies (Deschesnes, Couturier *et al.*, 2010) have shown that when the partnering sectors of school and health services do not understand and respect each other's core mission, the processes are not beneficial either to the health promotion process or to the school development in general.

Sustainability

Only two of the sources explicitly identified sustainability as a core component for implementation of health promoting schools (Aldinger *et al.*, 2008; Inchley *et al.*, 2007). Nevertheless, general implementation theory strongly advocates the importance of addressing sustainability from the very beginning of the implementation process. In this regard the school leadership is seen to have a key role (Fullan, 1992, 2001; Larsen & Samdal, 2008). According to Fullan (2005: ix) sustainability is 'the capacity of a system to engage in the complexities of

TABLE 4.2 Theoretically based rationale for the implementation components for health promoting schools

Implementation component	Aim of component	Theoretical base for component	Examples of literature for theoretical and empirical base
Preparing and planning for school development	Systematic planning identifying clear aims and priorities – taking into account the current situation and competence at school level, and consulting stakeholders – is vital to achieve sustainable change.	Goal commitment and collective efficacy Organisational change, school change and innovation	Bandura, 1998 Hopkins and Jackson, 2003 Heward et al., 2007
Policy and institutional anchoring	Inclusion of an intervention in policy documents and use of process to ensure institutional anchoring is likely to stimulate commitment in staff and help to prioritise resources for intervention. The anchoring processes using strategies of alignment are core to building readiness and organisational capacity.	Organisational change, school change and innovation Implementation theory	Hopkins and Jackson, 2003 Heward et al., 2007 Elias et al., 2003
Professional development and learning	Training in leadership and identified priority areas helps build motivation and competence for executive staff, the core team and other staff, essential for quality implementation of change.	Organisational change, educational change, adult learning principles (experiential)	Mihalic et al., 2004 Hopkins and Jackson, 2003 Heward et al., 2007 Easton, 2008 Fullan, 2008
Leadership and management practices	Leadership actions in building ownership in the school community and anchoring the activities to school visions through feedback, encouragement and expectations to implement actions are fundamental to maintain focus and motivation among stakeholders for agreed change.	Social learning theory, social cognitive theory, social support Leadership theory	Bandura, 1998 Farrell et al., 2001 Fullan, 2001, 2005, 2008 Kam et al., 2003 Leithwood et al., 2007

Relational and organisational context	The social relations and the structural conditions of a school can maximise the achievement of agreed actions by providing a stimulating climate and opportunities.	Social learning theory, social climate Organisational capacity	Bandura, 1998 McBride et al., 1999 Sabatier, 1997 Elias, 2003 Hopkins and Jackson, 2003 Flaspohler et al., 2008
Student participation	Student participation is a means and a goal to maximise motivation for health and learning. It values and provides conditions for them to be empowered.	Self-determination theory, agency, initiative, school connectedness Civic engagement Relational pedagogy	Ryan and Deci, 2000 Jensen and Simovska, 2005 Boyd et al., 2006
Partnerships and networking	Active parental involvement in a variety of ways can facilitate parental support for values and actions of the school. Involvement of relevant collaborators may stimulate action and commitment through complementary expertise and expectations.	Social learning theory Social climate Organisational capacity, including competence input from partners	Bandura, 1998 Deschesnes et al., 2003 Inchley et al., 2007 Hopkins and Jackson, 2003 Leurs et al., 2005 Boot et al., 2010
Sustainability	Long term maintenance of the initiative is dependent on a continued focus on conditions that facilitate and ensure implementation of agreed actions for change.	Implementation theory (institutionalisation and monitoring)	Hoelscher et al., 2004 Fullan, 2005, 2008 Inchley et al., 2007 Aldinger et al., 2008 Larsen and Samdal, 2008

Source: Samdal and Rowling, 2011, © Emerald Publishing Group, reprinted with permission

continuous improvement consistent with deep values of human purpose'. To ensure continuous follow-up of stakeholders it is necessary to check progress and priority of actions and activities. Thus self and group evaluations of current practice and activities will help the school to keep focus and identify the need for change or higher dose of efforts if little progress in health promotion perceptions is identified. The leadership may in this process also monitor action by asking stakeholders to report regularly on their activities and also invite them to discussion around implementation challenges to avoid having these stop the change progress. Previous research has identified that this balance of monitoring and support stimulates the desired change behaviour (Daft, 1999; Larsen & Samdal, 2008). It further demonstrates the continued support and commitment from the leadership to the change process of implementing the health promoting school policy. From a social learning theory perspective, this role modelling and prioritising might be important for the continued motivation and priority setting from the rest of the stakeholders (Bandura, 1998). Long term sustainability is also stimulated by other actions of institutionalisation, such as continued inclusion in policy documents, systematic professional development and learning for new staff, as well booster sessions for all staff and stable resource allocation (Hoelscher *et al.*, 2004). As already commented, sustainability needs to be addressed from the start of the implementation process. More specifically, it should be taken into consideration when working with each of the other seven implementation components to ensure a consistent focus of continuity.

Discussion

The eight implementation components for health promoting schools identified through the meta-analysis could be matched with the three cross cutting categories for change processes in school identified in the introduction. The cross cutting categories were building on strategies and components identified by Daft (1999), Hargreaves and colleagues (2001), and Hopkins and Jackson (2003) and include: (1) school leadership, (2) establishing readiness, and (3) organisational facilitation.

The first category of school leadership covers the two components of *Leadership and management* and *Policy and institutional anchoring*. The importance of supportive leadership for health promoting change processes in school is also highlighted by previous research (Tjomsland *et al.*, 2010; Tjomsland, Larsen, Viig & Wold, 2009; Weiner *et al.*, 2009). The role seems to cover both the leadership actions in terms of providing direction and support, as well as allocating funding. Moreover, the role of the leadership in ensuring policy and institutional anchoring through delegated leadership and inclusive decision making is advocated as this brings the stakeholders on board.

The second category of creating readiness can be seen to capture the components of *Planning and preparing for development, Professional development and learning,* and *Student participation.* The readiness approach is about providing direction and visions by identifying how the innovation fits with the overall values and aims of the school. This fit is frequently considered a prerequisite for implementation success (Weiner *et al.*, 2009). The approach is about preparing an organisation and the participants for their participation in implementation action (Elias *et al.*, 2003; Weiner *et al.*, 2009), represented by the actions specifically covered in the component of *Preparing and planning*. Further the *Professional development and learning* addresses development of competence for stakeholders to take part in the planned actions and will also assist in the alignment of teachers and other stakeholders to contribute to achieve the aims of the health promoting school policy. Student participation is also placed in this category as this involves giving students opportunities to influence both the planning and the implementation of actions. Their voice needs to be heard as to what priorities they think should be addressed. They also are likely to benefit from training in developing skills for providing input and operating in democratic discussions where they could meet different priorities and interests.

The third category addresses organisational facilitation and will naturally include the components of *Relational and organisational context, Partnerships and networking,* and *Sustainability*. These components are about structures and practices that enable the school to conduct the specific and needed actions. Relational and organisation context involves exchange of ideas and experiences among stakeholders as well as helping and motivating each other throughout the change process. Previous research has also identified the importance of mutual support for health promoting change processes in school (Viig & Wold, 2005), and the positive impact of an overall implementation climate addressing collaboration within school and networking with partners (Boot *et al.*, 2010; Leurs *et al.*, 2005). Finally the sustainability component is included here as it also represents a key organisational emphasis and willingness to follow up the intervention over time and thereby an important source of an initial and continued change process.

The identification of the implementation components as presented in this chapter and previously reported by Rowling and Samdal (2011) and Samdal and Rowling (2011) represents a unique approach to identify a comprehensive theoretical base for implementation of health promoting schools. A clear strength of the work is that the sources that are utilised for identifying the specific components build on data from different cultures. Further, each source had identified a minimum of five of the extracted implementation components. This provides a strong base for global application of the components despite differences in cultures and school systems.

It is clearly a limitation of the extraction of the components that they arise from analyses of only eight articles. This demonstrates the scarcity in the scientific reporting on implementation of health promoting schools. More research is essential to both test the applicability of the identified implementation components as well as further exploration for inclusion of other relevant components. The parameters for this are elaborated in Chapter 10.

Conclusions

While Daft (1999), Hargreaves and colleagues (2001) and Hopkins and Jackson (2003) have identified fairly broad categories of change processes in school, this chapter presents theory-driven implementation components for health promoting schools that provide greater specificity. It provides practitioners with more detailed guidelines, presenting opportunities for rigorous performance and fidelity to implement actions to meet the objectives of the health promoting school policy. A clear rationale is, however, not sufficient guidance for implementing the components with fidelity. Chapter 5 will therefore provide more details on how to more specifically implement the components, i.e. which concrete actions are needed.

Note

1   This chapter is based on the article by Samdal & Rowling (2011). Theoretical base for implementation components of health promoting schools. *Health Education*, *111*(5), 367–390. © Emerald Publishing Group

References

Aldinger, C., Zhang, X.-W., Liu, L.-Q., Guo, J.-X., Yu Sen Hai & Jones, J. (2008). Strategies for implementing Health-Promoting Schools in a province in China. *Promotion & Education*, *15*(1), 24–29.

Allensworth, D. D., Wyche, J., Lawson, E. & Nicholson, L. (1995). *Defining a Comprehensive School Health Program: An Interim Statement. Division of Health Sciences Policy.* Washington, DC: National Academy Press.

Bandura, A. (1998). Health promotion from the perspective of social cognitive theory. *Psychology & Health*, *13*(4), 623–649.

Barnekow, V., Buijs, G., Clift, S., Jensen, B. B., Paulus, P., Rivett, D. & Young, I. (2006). *Health-promoting Schools: A Resource for Developing Indicators.* Copenhagen: World Health Organization.

Bond, L., Glover, S., Godfrey, C., Butler, H. & Patton, G. C. (2001). Building Capacity for System-Level Change in Schools: Lessons from the Gatehouse Project. *Health Education & Behavior*, *28*(3), 368–383.

Boot, N., van Assama, P., Hesdal, B. & de Vries, N. (2010). Professional assistance in implementing school health policies. *Health Education*, *110*(4), 294–308.

Boyd, R., MacNeill, N. & Sullivan, G. (2006). Relational pedagogy: putting balance back into students' learning. *Curriculum Leadership*, *4*(13). www.curriculum.edu.au/leader/relational_pedagogy=putting_balance_back_into_stu,13944.html?issueID=10277 (accessed 25 September 2012).

Buijs, G. J. (2009). Better Schools through Health: networking for health promoting schools in Europe. *European Journal of Education*, *44*(4), 507–520.

Burgher, M., Rasmussen, V. B. & Rivett, D. (1999). *The European Network of Health Promoting Schools: The alliance of education and health.* Copenhagen: WHO.

Daft, R. L. (1999). *Leadership: Theory and Practice.* Fort Worth, TX: Dryden Press.

Danielsen, A. G., Samdal, O., Hetland, J. & Wold, B. (2009). School-related social support and students' perceived life satisfaction. *Journal of Educational Research, 102*(4), 303–318.

Darling-Hammond, L. (2009). Teaching and the change wars: the professionalism hypothesis. In A. Hargreaves & M. Fullan. (Eds), *Change Wars* (pp. 45–68). Bloomington, IN: Solution Tree.

Deci, E. L. & Ryan, R. M. (2000). The "what" and "why" of goal pursuits: human needs and the self-determination of behavior. *Psychological Inquiry, 11*(4), 227–268.

Denman, S. (1999). Health promoting schools in England – a way forward in development. *Journal of Public Health Medicine, 21*(2), 215–220.

Deschesnes, M., Couturier, Y., Laberge, S. & Campeau, L. (2010). How divergent conceptions among health and education stakeholders influence the dissemination of healthy schools in Quebec. *Health Promotion International, 25*(4), 435–443.

Deschesnes, M., Martin, C. & Hill, A. J. (2003). Comprehensive approaches to school health promotion: how to achieve broader implementation? *Health Promotion International, 18*(4), 387–396.

Deschesnes, M., Trudeau, F. & Kébé, M. (2010). Factors influencing the adoption of a Health Promoting School approach in the province of Quebec, Canada. *Health Education Research, 25*(3), 438–450.

Donaldson, G. A. (2001). *Cultivating Leadership in Schools: Connecting People, Purpose, and Practice.* New York: Teachers College Press.

Durlak, J. A. (2003). Generalizations regarding effective prevention and health promotion programs. In T. P. Gullotta & M. Bloom (Eds), *The Encyclopedia of Primary Prevention and Health Promotion* (pp. 61–69). New York: Kluwer Academic/Plenum.

Durlak, J. A. & DuPre, E. (2008). Implementation matters: a review of research on the influence of implementation on program outcomes and the factors affecting implementation. *American Journal of Community Psychology, 41*(3), 327–350.

Easton, L. B. (2008). From professional development to professional learning. *Phi Delta Kappa, 89*(10), 755–759.

Elias, M. J., Zins, J., Graczyk, P. & Weissberg, R. (2003). Implementation, sustainability, and scaling up of social-emotional and academic innovations in public schools. *School Psychology Review, 32*, 303–319.

Farrell, A. D., Meyer, A. L., Kung, E. M. & Sullivan, T. N. (2001). Development and Evaluation of School-Based Violence Prevention Programs. *Journal of Clinical Child & Adolescent Psychology, 30*(2), 207–220.

Felner, R. D., Favazza, A., Shim, M., Brand, S., Gu, K. & Noonan, N. (2001). Whole school improvement and restructuring as prevention and promotion lessons from STEP and the project on High Performance Learning Communities. *Journal of School Psychology, 39*(2), 177–202.

Flaspohler, P., Duffy, J., Wandersman, A., Stillman, L. & Maras, M. (2008). Unpacking Prevention Capacity: An Intersection of Research-to-practice Models and Community-centered Models. *American Journal of Community Psychology, 41*(3), 182–196.

Fullan, M. (1992). *Successful School Improvement.* Toronto, Canada: OISE Press.

Fullan, M. (2001). *Leading in a Culture of Change.* San Francisco, CA: Jossey-Bass.

Fullan, M. (2005). *Leadership and Sustainability. System Thinkers in Action.* Thousand Oaks, CA: Corwin Press.

Fullan, M. (2008). *The Six Secrets of Change. What the Best Leaders Do to Help Their Organizations Survive and Thrive.* San Fransisco, CA: Jossey-Bass.

Fullan, M., Cuttress, C. & Kilcher, A. (2009). Eight forces for leaders of change. In M. Fullan (Ed.), *The Challenge of Change. Start School Improvement Now!* (pp. 9–20). Thousand Oaks, CA: Corwin.

Fullan, M. & Huberman, M. (1992). *Successful School Improvement: The Implementation Perspective and Beyond.* Buckingham: Open University Press.

Green, L. W. & Kreuter, M. W. (2005). *Health Promotion Planning: An Educational and Ecological Approach* (4th edn). New York, NY: McGraw-Hill.

Guldbrandsson, K. & Bremberg, S. (2006). Two approaches to school health promotion – a focus on health-related behaviours and general competencies. An ecological study of 25 Swedish municipalities. *Health Promotion International, 21*(1), 37–44.

Hallinger, P. (2003). Leading Educational Change: reflections on the practice of instructional and transformational leadership. *Cambridge Journal of Education, 33*(3), 329–352.

Hargreaves, A., Earl, L., Moore, S. & Manning, S. (2001). *Learning to Change. Teaching Beyond Subjects and Standards.* San Francisco, CA: Jossey-Bass Inc.

Harris, A. & Lambert, L. (2003). *Building Leadership Capacity for School Improvement.* Maidenhead: Open University Press.

Hattie, J. (2009). *Visible learning. A Synthesis of over 800 Meta-Analyses Relating to Achievement.* Abingdon, Oxon: Routledge.

Heward, S., Hutchins, C. & Keleher, H. (2007). Organizational change – key to capacity building and effective health promotion. *Health Promotion International, 22*(2), 170–178.

Hoelscher, D. M., Feldman, H. A., Johnson, C. C., Lytle, L. A., Osganian, S. K., Parcel, G. S. *et al.* (2004). School-based health education programs can be maintained over time: results from the CATCH Institutionalization study. *Preventive Medicine, 38*(5), 594–606.

Holthe, A., Larsen, T. & Samdal, O. (2011). Implementation of national guidelines for healthy school meals: the relationship between process and outcome. *Scandinavian Journal of Educational Research, 55*(4), 357–378.

Hopkins, D. & Jackson, D. (2003). Building the capacity for leading and learning. In A. Harris (Ed.), *Effective Leadership for School Improvment.* New York: Teachers College Press.

Hoyle, T. B., Samek, B. B. & Valois, R. F. (2008). Building Capacity for the Continuous Improvement of Health-Promoting Schools. *Journal of School Health, 78*(1), 1–8.

Inchley, J., Muldoon, J. & Currie, C. (2007). Becoming a health promoting school: evaluating the process of effective implementation in Scotland. *Health Promotion International, 22*(1), 65–71.

Jensen, B. B. & Simovska, V. (2005). Involving students in learning and health promotion processes – clarifying what? how? and why? *Promotion & Education, 12*(3–4), 150–156.

Kallestad, J. H. & Olweus, D. (2003). Predicting teachers' and schools' implementation of the Olweus bullying prevention program: A multilevel study. *Prevention & Treatment, 6*(1), Article 21.

Kam, C.-M., Greenberg, M. T. & Walls, C. T. (2003). Examining the role of implementation quality in school-based prevention using the PATHS curriculum. *Prevention Science, 4*(1), 55–63.

Larson, R. (2000). Towards a psychology of positive youth development. *American Psychologist, 55*(1), 170–183.

Larsen, T. & Samdal, O. (2007). Implementing second step: balancing fidelity and program adaptation. *Journal of Educational and Psychological Consultation, 17*(1), 1–29.

Larsen, T. & Samdal, O. (2008). Facilitating the Implementation and sustainability of second step. *Scandinavian Journal of Educational Research, 52*(2), 187–204.

Leithwood, K., Mascall, B., Strauss, T., Sacks, R., Memon, N. & Yashkina, A. (2007). Distributing leadership to make schools smarter: taking the ego out of the system. *Leadership and Policy in Schools*, *6*(1), 37–67.

Leurs, M. T. W., Schaalma, H. P., Jansen, M. W. J., Mur-Veeman, I. M., St. Leger, L. H. & de Vries, N. (2005). Development of a collaborative model to improve school health promotion in the Netherlands. *Health Promotion International*, *20*(3), 296–305.

McBride, N. (2000). The Western Australian School Health Project: comparing the effects of intervention intensity on organizational support for school health promotion. *Health Education Research*, *15*(1), 59–72.

McBride, N., Midford, R. & Cameron, I. (1999). An empirical model for school health promotion: the Western Australian school health project model. *Health Promotion International*, *14*(1), 17–25.

McGraw, S. A., Sellers, D., Stone, E., Resnicow, K. A., Kuester, S., Fridinger, F. & Wechsler, H. (2000). Measuring implementation of school programs and policies to promote healthy eating and physical activity among youth. *Preventive Medicine: An International Journal Devoted to Practice and Theory*, *31*(2, Pt. 2), S86–S97.

Mihalic, S., Irwin, K., Fagan, A., Ballard, D. & Eliott, D. (2004). Successful Program Implementation: Lessons From Blueprints. *Juvenile Justice Bulletin*, July, 1–11.

Neil, P., McEwen, A., Carlisle, K. & Knipe, D. (2001). The self-evaluating school – a case study of a special school. *British Journal of Special Education*, *28*(4), 174–181.

Parsons, C., Stears, D. & Thomas, C. (1996). The health promoting school in Europe: conceptualising and evaluating the change. *Health Education Journal*, *55*(3), 311–321.

Reeve, J. & Jang, H. (2006). What teachers say and do to support students' autonomy during learning activities. *Journal of Educational Psychology*, *98*, 209–218.

Rogers, E. M. (2003). *Diffusion of Innovations*. New York: Free Press.

Rowling, L. & Samdal, O. (2011). Filling the black box of implementation for health-promoting schools. *Health Education*, *111*(5), 347–366.

Ryan, R. M. & Deci, E. L. (2000). Self-determination theory and the facilitation of intrinsic motivation, social development, and well-being. *American Psychologist*, *55*(1), 68–78.

Sabatier, P. A. (1997). Top–down and bottom–up approaches to implementation research. In M. Hill (Ed.), *The Policy Process: A Reader* (2nd edn, pp. 272–295). Harlow: Pearson/Harvester Wheatsheaf.

Samdal, O. (2008). School health promotion. In H. Heggenhougen (Ed.), *The Encyclopedia of Public Health* (Vol. 5, pp. 653–661). Oxford: Elsevier Inc.

Samdal, O., Nutbeam, D., Wold, B. & Kannas, L. (1998). Achieving health and educational goals through schools: A study of the importance of school climate and students' satisfaction with school. *Health Education Research*, *13*(3), 383–397.

Samdal, O. & Rowling, L. (2011). Theoretical and empirical base for implementation components of health promoting schools. *Health Education*, *3*(5), 367–390.

Samdal, O., Viig, N. G. & Wold, B. (2010). Health promotion integrated into school policy and practice: experiences of implementation in the Norwegian network of health promoting schools. *Journal of Child and Adolescent Psychology*, *1*(2), 43–72.

Samdal, O., Wold, B., and Bronis, M. (1999): The relationship between students' perceptions of the school environment, their satisfaction with school and perceived academic achievement: an international study. *School Effectiveness and School Improvement*, *10*(3), 296–320.

Senge, P. (2006). *The Fifth Discipline: The Art and Practice of the Learning Organization* (2nd edn). New York: Doubleday.

Stefanou, C. R., Perencevich, K. C., DiCintio, M., and Turner, J. C. (2004). Supporting autonomy in the classroom: Ways teachers encourage student decision making and ownership. *Educational Psychologist*, *39*, 97–110.

Stith, S., Pruitt, I., Dees, J., Fronce, M., Green, N., Som, A. & Linkh, D. (2006). Implementing community-based prevention programming: a review of the literature. *The Journal of Primary Prevention*, *27*(6), 599–617.

Thomas, C., Parsons, C. & Stears, D. (1998). Implementing the European network of health promoting schools in Bulgaria, the Czech Republic, Lithuania and Poland: vision and reality. *Health Promotion International*, *13*(4), 329–338.

Tjomsland, H. E., Larsen, T. M. B., Samdal, O. & Wold, B. (2010). Sustaining comprehensive physical activity practice in elementary school: A case study applying mixed methods. *Teachers and Teaching: Theory and Practice*, *16*(1), 73–95.

Tjomsland, H. E., Larsen, T. M. B., Viig, N. G. & Wold, B. (2009). A fourteen-year follow-up study of health promoting schools in Norway: principals' perceptions of conditions influencing sustainability. *The Open Education Journal*, *2*, 54–64.

Viig, N. G., Tjomsland, H. E. & Wold, B. (2010). Program and school characteristics related to teacher participation in school health promotion. *The Open Education Journal*, *3–11*(10–20).

Viig, N. G. & Wold, B. (2005). Facilitating teachers' participation in school-based health promotion – a qualitative study. *Scandinavian Journal of Educational Research*, *49*(1), 83–109.

Weiner, B. J., Lewis, M. A. & Linnan, L. A. (2009). Using organization theory to understand the determinants of effective implementation of worksite health promotion programs. *Health Education Research*, *24*(2), 292–305.

5

THEORY AND EMPIRICALLY-BASED IMPLEMENTATION OF ELEMENTS IN COMPONENTS[1]

Louise Rowling and Oddrun Samdal

Introduction

Previous chapters have articulated the debates, perspectives and challenges faced in quality whole school implementation to create health promoting schools. They have established that the 'science of delivery' (Catford, 2009) in this field has not yet been articulated, despite the recognition by educational researchers that fidelity of implementation of an innovation is an essential factor to monitor and document because it helps explain the outcomes (Dusenbury, Brannigan, Falco & Hansen, 2003). Eight components of implementation have been described in the previous chapter based on a meta-analysis (or literature review) of theory and empirical work (Samdal & Rowling, 2011). However, it is not sufficient merely to identify these components, it is essential also to provide specificity within these components for quality practice in implementation. The specificity of elements of the components delineated here arises from organisational, implementation and educational theories and empirical work. From this literature, elements for action can be established that are firmly anchored in existing research and cumulatively build each component. They function as mechanisms (activities and procedures within a context) (Whitelaw, Martin, Kerr & Wimbush, 2006) that can operationalise the interplay of the individual and the organisation in organisational change, assist to achieve quality practice and guide evaluation (see Figure 5.1).

While the components are examined separately in this chapter, it is important to recognise that implementation involves an integrated set of components (Deschesnes *et al.*, 2010). Additionally there are underpinning implementation conditions that have already been elaborated. These practice based conditions include culture and context (Flaspohler, Duffy, Wandersman, Stillman & Maras, 2008; Hargreaves, Earl, Moore & Manning, 2001), state of readiness of the

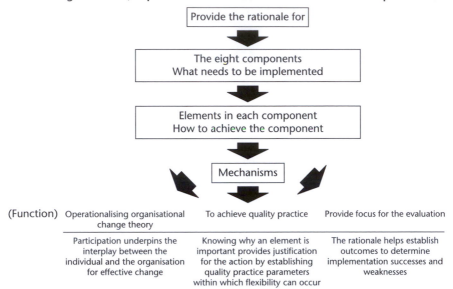

Organisational, implementation and educational theories and empirical work

Provide the rationale for

The eight components
What needs to be implemented

Elements in each component
How to achieve the component

Mechanisms

(Function)	Operationalising organisational change theory	To achieve quality practice	Provide focus for the evaluation
	Participation underpins the interplay between the individual and the organisation for effective change	Knowing why an element is important provides justification for the action by establishing quality practice parameters within which flexibility can occur	The rationale helps establish outcomes to determine implementation successes and weaknesses

FIGURE 5.1   Framework articulating the relationship between the research, the implementation components and their elements

organisation (Elias, Zins, Graczyk & Weissberg, 2003; Flaspohler *et al.*, 2008; Weiner, Lewis & Linnan, 2009), leadership within education and health (Hoyle, Samek & Valois, 2008; Rowling & Mason, 2005; Tjomsland, Iversen & Wold, 2009). Favourable conditions help build the capacity of individuals and organisations, an essential feature of the health promoting school, and establish that participation underpins the interplay between the individual and the organisation for effective change as outlined in Chapter 3.

Theoretical and empirical base for specificity of implementation

The previous chapter identifies the evidence base for eight components of implementation of health promoting schools. However, to ensure quality in the implementation process, a theoretical and empirical evidence base is also needed for how the components should operate. The identification of an evidence base for an implementation system for health promoting schools signifies that it is not just the existence of the components to which attention needs to be paid, but also their functioning as a key outcome to be achieved (Rowling & Samdal, 2011). Recording the functioning of the implementation components, often labelled process evaluation, as a means to achieve desired outcomes is intended to provide a new focus for strengthening the science base for health promoting schools, as has been repeatedly called for over the past decade (Deschesnes, Martin & Hill,

2003; Lister-Sharp *et al.*, 1999; Stewart-Brown, 2006). Table 5.1 exemplifies elements of how to implement each component, the rationale for each element and organisational, implementation, and educational theories and empirical sources that provide the rationale for specific elements. For example, when a core team is being developed, trainers and practitioners will know why this is important and can easily access the theoretical and empirical bases in the references that provide further elaboration.

Preparing and planning for school development

Dür argues in a previous chapter in this text that the socio–economic pressures on countries globally require further development of schools as the central organisation of modern education systems (Dür, Chapter 3 above). Educational research reflects this focus on whole school development rather than piecemeal attention to separate sections of school life. For example, a focus on 'the whole child' might be implemented by focusing on child centred teaching methods. This ignores both the social disadvantage conditions that might impact on the learning, health and well-being of children in the school, and the limited resources that may be available to teachers in areas of social disadvantage. The impact of these conditions means that the local situation can hamper or facilitate change and whole school development. These conditions need to be identified within each school. Achieving this needs preparation so that action can be targeted to address setting specific conditions of the school, as the planning for programme, policy or service is implemented (see discussion Barry and Dooris, Chapter 2 above). In preparing for implementation, cognisance of local conditions includes identifying existing policies, goals, structures and practices supporting the aims of health promoting schools initiatives, thereby stimulating the anchoring of the approach in the existing school organisation (Green & Kreuter, 2005; Samdal, Viig & Wold, 2010). This situation is different from many initiatives where the implementation involves existing interventions which the organisation has agreed to implement, often without modification to suit the local conditions. A process of organisational change and school development is therefore integral to creating health promoting schools (Heward, Hutchins & Keleher, 2007) and requires preparation and planning.

Readiness is a key action element in preparing for organisational change in schools. It may be a precursor to school based planning or a parallel process. Using existing research literature, Flaspohler and colleagues (2008) identified a set of factors that indicate schools might be ready for change. These were:

- *Ability*: the resources and capabilities of the school and community;
- *Values*: the degree to which the change fits with the school and community vision and operations;
- *Idea*: the clarity and understandability of the change to the school and community;

- *Circumstances:* features of the school and community environment that make it easier or harder to make the change;
- *Timing:* the readiness of the school and community to consider the change, especially in relation to other school improvement efforts;
- *Obligation:* the felt need to change or 'do something different';
- *Resistances:* inhibiting factors in the school and community that act against the change;
- *Yield:* perceived benefits of the change.

An empirical study in Australia in the mid-1990s illustrates the key role of readiness in implementation. A 22-month research project developed two 'readiness' scales, school organisational support and school health promotion. Their results showed that teacher professional development acted as a catalyst for school based organisational change and that this could occur within the time of the study and be sustained for at least a year. However, the school health promotion change was not evident until a year after the intervention, leading researchers to conclude that organisational change was a precursor to implementation of health promotion. The readiness step in the planning process is an essential action area requiring time and energy for developing preparedness in organisations and gaining commitment from school personnel. Additionally, establishing commitment from the leadership can be facilitated by incorporating the proposed actions in the school's policy plan as well as by identifying resources for the initiative (Sabatier, 1997).

As outlined previously (Samdal & Rowling, 2011; Dür, Chapter 3 above), a core element of a health promoting school is the involvement of all the participants in the organisation in identification of an area that needs change and strategies or actions that can help the organisation achieve the needed change. Readiness of the organisation can begin the process of ensuring that the voices of all relevant participants are heard. The establishment of a coordination committee with representatives from all relevant stakeholders in the school (staff, students, parents, and others) can assist this. While establishing a coordination committee has been recommended practice (Denman, 1999) it is not just the existence of the committee that is important but its functioning and representation of all stakeholders' perspectives. An Australian student well-being research project found that action teams that were successful in their implementation phase had similarities including regular meetings in school time, inclusion of leadership personnel, retention of most of the team members over at least three years, drawing members from a broad base within the school, and having clearly defined roles and shared team responsibility, rather than leaving most of the work to one or two people. Team member qualities that helped in the successful implementation included perseverance and dedication in following up responsibilities despite difficulties and other commitments, organisational ability, collegial respect, flexibility, ability to assume authority and to delegate (Firth *et al.*, 2008).

Programme theory based planning can help guide work, e.g. Program Logic (Kellogg Foundation, 2004); or Green and Kreuter's (2005) planning model for health promotion that identifies all steps that need to be taken. These models focus on the functioning of components and accommodate unique and dynamic contexts. An examination of these planning models provides greater detail for action. For example Green and Kreuter identify three main elements in the planning of actions: (i) needs assessment, (ii) prioritise needs, and (iii) identify actions to meet needs.

In identifying actions to meet the agreed needs or aims for the intervention it is of importance to begin by searching for existing programmes or approaches which can be used to meet the identified need and which have demonstrated effectiveness. A pre-package programme frequently builds on theory with identified mechanisms to achieve the desired change. Examples of such pre-package programmes or strategies are Olweus' anti-bullying programme (Olweus, 1993) for schools that have identified that they want to reduce bullying, or the programme on anxiety and depression for schools (Lowry-Webster et al., 2003) that aims to address mental illness. If no such programme is available, the school needs to devise activities and actions themselves that can help them meet their identified need.

Another planning model involves developing programme logic frameworks. In a programme logic model a causal pathway is created by specifying the elements of a programme and by identifying 'if . . . then . . .' relationships (Kellogg Foundation, 2004). The process of thinking through the relationships between elements being utilised enables assumptions that link the components to be made more explicit (Patton, 2004). The causal relationships between elements may be affected (positively or negatively) by key contextual factors such as funding cycles that impact on the programme but that cannot be controlled.

A crucial element in the planning phase is also to make an evaluation plan. Ideally a baseline survey should be conducted and later followed up to see if the actions have contributed to change. This could focus on identifying the frequency of the identified behaviour or the perceptions or knowledge that need to change. Moreover, student and staff approval of the activities are relevant to assess as this will be important for their motivation and commitment to participate in the activities. It is also recommended that the coordination committee plan for actions that maximise sustainability, from the very beginning of the project. Such actions relate, for instance, to long-term anchoring of the initiate in policy plans and ongoing resources for professional development (Larsen & Samdal, 2008; Sabatier, 1997).

Policy and institutional anchoring

A key strategy for school change for improved health outcomes is the development and/or review of school/district level policies (Deschesnes et al., 2003; Samdal, 2008). Policies can provide a vision, a mandate, decisions and actions, a strategy for action and support through the specification of the provision of financial, organisational and technical resources (Daft, 1999). Also, written policy clearly communicates to existing and new school community members a scaffold for school development, especially when part of the school vision is articulated as 'creating a health promoting school' (Bond, Glover, Godfrey, Butler & Patton, 2001; Hoyle *et al.*, 2008). Establishing commitment from the leadership can be facilitated by incorporating the proposed actions in the school's policy plan as well as by identifying resources for the initiative (Sabatier, 1997).

In a review of the Norwegian Network of Health Promoting Schools, it was found that policy included both cross-curricular plans for health education and objectives for the psychosocial school environment. Several of the teachers emphasised that the important function of the policy document was to maintain focus, secure continuity and commit new teachers to present priorities at the school (Samdal *et al.*, 2010).

In a wider societal perspective, national and state political and financial support exemplified through public policy is essential for action in all health promotion (Leeder, 1997). This is particularly important for the complexity of intersectoral settings approaches.

Professional development and learning

Acknowledging the importance of the interplay of individuals with organisational factors in schools is necessary as school personnel are key initiators of change (Samdal, 2008). Professional development increases teacher capacity for action and, linked with school-based professional learning, contributes to building teacher efficacy for active involvement. Within this, development of competencies is a key outcome. This does not involve developing a skill in isolation, but designates the knowledge of how to act in a particular situation with a specific set of constraints and resources, that is, successful action in a specific context (Jourdan, 2011). Teachers can only be deemed competent after they have dealt with a particular situation and when the actions are considered socially acceptable (Jonnaert, Barrette & Masciotra, 2006). This action in context is professional learning.

Distinguishing between professional development and professional learning is important for effective capacity building. Professional development often takes place off the school premises and can involve external networking. It is usually decided upon by people from above (a top-down approach) and focuses primarily on knowledge and competency development and occasionally consideration of attitudes. By contrast, professional learning is school based (a bottom-up approach), and focuses on knowledge, attitudes, skills, aspirations and behaviour (Easton, 2008). Professional learning is embedded in the work that teachers do and can occur in a variety of ways: school-based conversations, observing and being coached, mentoring, analysing and planning individually and groupwork (Easton, 2008).

An example of the interconnection of this professional development and professional learning occurred in the implementation of the Australian national mental health promotion resource materials MindMatters. Teachers were actively engaged in contributing to the development of the materials. As they experienced the professional development and then used materials for school based training with their staff, they provided feedback to the project team about the need to address the crucial role of a teacher's personal engagement with mental health and the sensitive nature of the area. The result was a consultative developmental process where the school-based professional learning provided feedback to the offsite professional development (Mason & Rowling, 2005). An outcome of this process was that more development time was identified as being needed to look at the emotional intelligence aspects of teaching; teaching styles and self efficacy; and examining attitudes and beliefs towards health and well-being. These elements were critical to teachers' and other education staff's resilience, happiness and longevity in their role (Mason & Rowling, 2005). That is, in the MindMatters programme training reflected and modelled the material being promoted and took care to respect the professionalism of teachers providing development both in educational terms and as individuals learning and working in a school (Rowling & Mason, 2005). The evaluation of the professional development established the training as a key element in improving teacher efficacy for mental health and wellbeing (Rowling, 2009; Rowling & Samdal, 2011).

While many reports on health projects with schools include reference to change agents, mentors, coaches, advisors, critical friends or, more often, a facilitator (Bond et al., 2001), little elaboration of the role is found. One study elaborated the role of school health promotion advisors in the Schoolbeat programme in the Netherlands (Boot, van Assama, Hesdal & de Vries, 2010). Competencies that were identified as needed by these advisors included knowledge of health promotion activities, social skills, a feeling of mutual understanding and the ability to plan. Acquiring these diverse skills and competencies needs ongoing training, coaching and professional learning within the context of schools as well as acquisition of knowledge of research on educational change and innovation. The evaluators of the programme found that both assistance to schools and building trust in relationships were essential in the success of the school health promotion advisor's role. Their role must be a collaborative one of a critical friend, not solely a technical giving of information.

Further elaboration on being a critical friend in the school development process describes the role as being dynamic, requiring a high level of skill and flexibility or, as one author described, 'I watch, I listen, I question, I wait . . . I do less of the doing and more of the directing and allowing' Butler et al. (2011: 12). To carry out this role critical friends need support to be able to:

- hold firm to a project's conceptual framework;
- step back and review progress and regain perspective;
- reconnect with the purpose of the project;
- regain professional perspective;
- theorise and draw lessons from common experiences;

- make visible what has become invisible;
- maintain energy, motivation and creativity;
- not take things personally;
- deal with challenges.

(Butler *et al.*, 2011: 14).

These supportive conditions create an environment for reflexive practice empowering participants, creating a learning community, readiness and commitment.

It is vitally important to monitor the role of the critical friend as, without some clear support, great variation in implementation can occur. The evaluation of the National Healthy Schools Programme in England, identified differences in the way local coordinators saw their roles (Barnard *et al.*, 2009). Coordinators articulated their role as being helpful and supportive but not to pressurise; to help and challenge them to meet criteria; to ensure schools met certain standards; and to encourage schools to use the programme as a form of continuous improvement. The importance of close attention to professional development and learning is clear. If ignored evaluation is compromised.

Leadership and management practice

An important but frequently misunderstood element of the context of the school is leadership. Sometimes those in leadership positions, because of day to day demands, focus principally on management and administrative roles, with little time left to attend to leadership actions of aligning initiatives with the visions and aims of the school. Moreover, the concept of leadership is often narrowly defined as applying to the principal. Using both leadership and management strategies has been found to be vital to ensure the support context of the implementation (Daft, 1999; Fullan, 1992; Larsen & Samdal, 2008). A study of school development for health promoting schools found that if there was a focus on pedagogical development and general school development, more systematic approaches were likely to occur (Samdal *et al.*, 2010). Important processes that have been identified include sound decision making, effective human resource management, explicating a moral purpose, understanding change processes, relationship building, knowledge building, and coherence making (Fullan, 2005b). Schools need many leaders at many levels (Fullan, 2005b) for policy development, pedagogy, curriculum development, as well as partnership formation with parents and service providers. This 'distributed' leadership is seen as important for whole school innovation and is essential to achieve systemic change (Rowling, 2009) and teacher efficacy (Inchley, Muldoon & Currie, 2007). Fullan (2008: 55) argued that it is not just modelling leadership, but modelling how to develop other leaders by 'fostering coalescing leadership in which combinations of leaders work together'. This combination includes students, teachers and other educational personnel, parents and caregivers as well as outside service providers (Rowling, 2009). In schools such a group 'creates a special leadership body to own the linked visions for innovation and systemic change and to guide and support the change' (Center for Mental Health and Schools, 2006: 11).

In a settings based approach to health, the concept of distributed leadership (Spillane, 2006) is particularly valuable in understanding school participation and ownership, a key element previously identified in this chapter in the preparing and planning component. What differs here is not what is done but how. While the ultimate responsibility of the positional leader remains, it is how the leadership role is enacted that differs. Distributed leadership with school staff and the principal involved in decision making encourages and strengthens relational behaviour (Rowling & Samdal, 2011).

School management is a shared responsibility that operates in an open and collaborative style (Scottish Health Promoting Schools Unit, 2004). Focusing on a whole school approach, management is responsive to people and changing circumstances providing opportunities for stakeholders' contributions to decision making. Through the planning process detailed earlier in this chapter, good practice is monitored and action initiated to attain standards of achievement agreed with stakeholders in both health and education.

Relational and organisational support context

Implementation operates in a political context. The national implementation stage of the Australian MindMatters suite of programmes (Rowling & Mason, 2005) occurred at a time of shifting national policy that involved short funding cycles. This made a significant difference to the implementation that could be employed, the ongoing stability of staff within the project, the status of the project and therefore support from education systems and sectors and schools (Rowling & Samdal, 2011).

As highlighted in the policy and institutional anchoring section, it is important to ensure that the health promoting school approach is written into the school's policy plan. However, translating this policy to the classroom can be challenging. As exemplified in a previous section, an important area in the change process for the development of health promoting schools is pedagogic leadership (Rowling & Samdal, 2011). The relational behaviour within classrooms has been labelled relational pedagogy, practice that treats relationships as the foundation of good pedagogy (Boyd, MacNeill & Sullivan, 2006). It equips learners to become partners in their own education for life. At the same time, it recognises that building relationships without improved student learning across all of the dimensions of education does not constitute good pedagogy. Relational pedagogy suggests three key practices: reflective behaviours, class meetings, and student-centred learning (Boyd et al., 2006). An example of students as active participants in their learning is 'action competence' championed by Jensen and colleagues in Denmark (Jensen & Simovska, 2005). A study in China found that improved relationships were achieved in the health promoting schools implementation between teachers and students and between students and their parents (Aldinger *et al.*, 2008).

It is vital to look into physical and organisational structures that may promote effective implementation. For instance, if priority is given to the increase of physical activity in students, it is important that the physical environment of the school invites being physically active through its natural and built design. Moreover, if an identified need is to increase the psychosocial climate of the school through increased collaborative effort between staff and among students, it is vital that there are opportunities for coordination. This can be through organisational actions such as suitable timetabling and elimination of inessential meetings, supporting the collaboration of teachers with common professional learning goals. Insights gained from individual or group professional learning should also be disseminated through the school, and processes need to be established to ensure that this occurs (Cole, 2008; Rowling & Samdal, 2011).

Developing good relationships with parents is important. Parents as key partners rarely describe information from the school solely in terms of what is being communicated, they also describe it in terms of how it makes them feel as parents. They see school-to-home communication as an indicator of their relationship with schools. For example, if the communication is warm, friendly, comprehensive and jargon-free, parents perceive that the school welcomes them, is inclusive and values their role in their children's education. If information or communication is dogmatic and aloof, sparing in content, or not easily comprehended, parents feel that the school views them less positively or undervalues their role in schooling (Cuttance & Stokes, 2000).

Partnership and networking

Partnerships have been found to be difficult to develop in health promoting schools and require effective collaborative models (Samdal *et al.*, 2010). For effective partnerships, collaborations between school and community are needed that complement and enhance each other and evolve into comprehensive, integrated approaches (Center for Mental Health and Schools, 2008). Effective school partnerships involve:

- a sharing of power, responsibility and ownership, with each party having different roles;
- a degree of mutuality, that includes listening to each other and responsive dialogue;
- shared aims and goals based on a common understanding of health and educational needs of children;
- a commitment to joint action in which parents, students, teachers and health personnel work together.

(Cuttance & Stokes, 2000)

Moving towards partnership building and networking through policies and systemic change processes helps address the fragmentation of programmes and services that frequently evolves with health sector agencies, and provides opportunities for greater participation by parents. In reporting the case studies of two disadvantaged primary schools in Ireland, Clarke and colleagues (Clarke, O'Sullivan & Barry, 2010) found that the two schools provided very different contexts in terms of parent involvement. One school, designated as having the most serious disadvantage rating, had very low levels of parental engagement while the other was described as 'close-knit' with families involved with the school. The higher level of involvement parent group had a longer history and familiarity with collaborating with school members. This context of enhanced state of partnerships could be built upon in their subsequent health promoting school activities, maximising positive outcomes.

Developing effective partnerships requires stakeholder readiness, an enlightened vision, financial support, geographic space, creative leadership, effective working relationships, training, time and new multi-faceted roles for professionals. Clearly defined roles and institutional infrastructure are also needed, not just personal connections (Center for Mental Health and Schools, 2008). Hoyle and colleagues (2008: 512) outline key areas for activity including bringing together teams from several schools; providing adequate time for most of a school community to work together in individual school teams; involving the principal's participation with the team; providing cutting edge ideas central to the context of the changes to be made; and introducing a process for change that includes analysing conditions in the school, devising strategies for improvement, and developing plans to involve the rest of the school community in the change process (Rowling & Samdal, 2011).

In a Canadian study two methods were used to assess stakeholders' positions about Healthy Schools and how this affected dissemination (Deschesnes et al., 2010). Interviews were undertaken with key informants selected because of their role in dissemination of Healthy Schools in Quebec, and document analysis was conducted of policies published in 2000–2007. The study identified lack of strategies for effective communication, differences in conceptualisations, and leadership capacity being more visible at regional and local levels than at a national level. Along with these strategies, building trust (Boot et al., 2010) is a key principle that has been identified to underpin partnership development, in terms of participation and empowerment. Operating in an empowering way involves engaging participants such as students and parents to build their existing capacities and strengths and to enhance their sense of control (Inchley et al., 2007; Jensen & Simovska, 2005). One outcome of lack of participation of all stakeholders has been poor adoption (Boot et al., 2010), or difficulties in taking pilot programmes to scale. The Australian MindMatters model of development and implementation did not encounter this gap in the development phase, nor was it experienced in the dissemination, as there was ongoing co-operation between the developers, evaluators and practitioners (Rowling, 2008).

Recent education sector research has also explored capacity building and networking of schools. Lateral capacity building across schools occurs where principals and teacher leaders collaborate with other schools, to learn from and contribute to school improvement (Fullan, 2005a). Linking with local agencies, parents and other community resources can enhance outcomes (Rowling & Samdal, 2011).

Student participation

Classroom pedagogy has shifted in the past three decades to a more student-centred approach. This involves not only designing specific classroom activities for student interaction with the topic, their teacher and their peers, but also their active engagement in deciding the form and depth of learning. Engagement involves developing action competence in students to act to bring about positive changes. This engagement of students in learning has spread to include a wider engagement in the governance and decision making in the school. In some countries this has been limited to consulting students, but in others it has involved providing training and opportunity for student leadership and active participation (Holdsworth & Blanchard, 2006). This changed pedagogy and listening to student voices underpins the empowerment and capacity building of students. To be an empowering process, participation needs to help young people to learn that they can make a difference for themselves and for others (Jensen & Simovska, 2005). Research from the Netherlands identified that student support is linked to the likelihood and intensity of teacher engagement in the teaching of health (Leurs, Bessems, Schaalma & de Vries, 2007). Although this finding relates to classroom based implementation of health issues, rather than student participation as an integral part of health promoting schools, it highlights the impact of student involvement on teacher behaviour change for implementation of health teaching (Rowling & Samdal, 2011).

Factors involved in implementing effective participation include: selection, recruitment, and retention of youth, level of participation, organisational capacity and shifts in attitudes of both students and adults (Norman, 2001). Consultations with young people have revealed that youth participation models need to use an age appropriate model so that young people develop a sense of control, a sense of connectedness, and gain a sense of meaning that matches their cognitive and social skill levels. These key factors help in the development of responsibility and a degree of ownership of a project and assist to maintain youth participation (Australian Infant Child Adolescent and Family Mental Health Association, 2008). Young people vary in their interests, skills and confidence so multiple strategies and flexible approaches are needed, to enable young people to participate meaningfully. Any model developed needs to ensure an inclusive, non-judgmental approach so that one form of participation is not perceived as superior to another.

Simovska (2008) argues for the recognition of the role of participation as a contributing factor in student development, as it assists students in dealing with the complexities of their lives and the world they inhabit and in experiencing personal meaningful learning. Participation can occur through a range of processes and activities such as investigations and problem solving to expand students' ways of knowing (Rowling & Samdal, 2011).

Sustainability

Sustainability involves building the capacity of an organisation and individuals to move beyond thinking about a time limited project, to reflecting on how new approaches and practices can be built into school priorities. Failure to adopt this perspective can contribute to fragmentation of efforts (Center for Mental Health in Schools, 2008). Sustainability is a cross cutting issue through all the components. Actions to facilitate sustainability include long term anchoring of the initiative in a policy plan, ongoing resources for professional development, monitoring performance of agreed actions and evaluating progress (Larsen & Samdal, 2008; Sabatier, 1997). These are considered core elements in keeping a focus on and prioritising initiatives over time (Daft, 1999). Evaluation will also be an important indicator of whether the actions carried out were implemented in accordance with the plan and are producing the intended results. If successful implementation has been achieved, a new cycle of identifying priorities while maintaining the first, can be initiated. Less effort is likely to be needed for this new stage, if the previous actions have been sustained. The school will at this time be able to build on their experience from previous planning and implementation, and may thus be able to initiate new actions more quickly.

For sustainability, it is also important, to support continued professional learning and development, and to expand the number of staff with a common vision and competencies in performing agreed actions. Through maintaining focus on professional learning and development for existing as well as new staff, a steady and positive alignment process, where the majority of staff are working towards performing the agreed action or change, may be ensured. This means that continued allocation of resources, both for ongoing and for new activities, must be given priority. For sustainability it is important to evaluate the professional learning of staff. This needs to be done on a number of levels (Easton, 2008). The first is teacher behaviour, how teachers change the way they work to take action to create health promoting schools. As well as teacher behaviour change, the behaviour of school administrators can also be monitored as an indicator of systemic change. Equally, changed behaviour and raised levels of mutual trust in partnerships should also be examined. If the professional learning is occurring then it should also be possible to look for change in student behaviour (Easton, 2008; Rowling & Samdal, 2011).

Sustainability for education audiences of the Australian MindMatters implementation occurred through confirmation of the links between mental health and educational gains for students (Rowling & Mason, 2005). This link is a key factor of sustainability for all health actions. For example, the evaluators of

MindMatters implementation had to develop strategies that were respectful of schools, minimised disruption to school procedures, and maintained goodwill over an extended time period (Hazell, Vincent, Waring & Lewin, 2002). In order to sustain the effort required by schools over a four-year period and minimise evaluation fatigue, the evaluation process needed to be seen as a partnership in acquiring 'mutually interesting data' (Hazell *et al.*, 2002: 26).

The rationale for application of components

Table 5.1 portrays the linkage between the theoretical and empirical research about the elements along with their rationale. The rationale assists in indicating the breadth of the scope of an element and is a central focus for practitioners in identifying the flexibility parameters. They can choose to implement the element by using an action similar to that described in the rationale. Additionally, the rationale will constitute an important basis for identifying implementation success or weaknesses by evaluating if the described outcomes were achieved, for example whether involving a core team did impact on whole school commitment (Rowling & Samdal, 2011).

Conclusions

In identifying and operationalising components for implementation for health promoting schools, attention needs to be paid to the existing research on the barriers and hindrances to implementation (Barry, Domitrovich & Lara, 2005; Deschesnes *et al.*, 2003).

The level of specificity provided in this chapter should enhance staff professional learning as it fulfils one of the characteristics for successful school based change, namely practical, detailed implementation and enough flexibility to allow shaping to suit to specific contexts (Cole, 2008). In the past the 'how' to implement whole school change was left to the variable knowledge and skills of practitioners involved in health promoting schools, resulting in disparity in amount and type of implementation, thereby contributing to differing outcomes. The absence of specific guidelines for implementation has hampered the development of rigour in the implementation and evaluation of health promoting schools.

The articulation of evidence based components for implementation detailed in this chapter is a significant step forward for health promoting schools. The specificity provided here holds promise to enhance the science base and quality of implementation. The implementation components detailed now need to be tested by schools and researchers for fit with content and contexts. Global testing of the components will expand knowledge on the social and geopolitical factors that impact on implementation. However, action will need to continue to highlight the links between education and health.

It could be argued that creating health promoting schools is an 'implementation approach', yet this has until now never been articulated.

TABLE 5.1 Summary of theoretically and empirically–based rationale of how to apply the implementation components for health promoting schools

How to implement the components	Why/rationale for how	Examples of literature for theoretical and empirical base
Preparing and planning for school development • Establish a core team and hold regular meetings • Consult with and survey the stakeholders, establishing their level of readiness • Analyse data and negotiate two or three priority areas for change • Set goals that reflect the needs and capacities of the school within realistic timelines using a planning tool such as Program Logic • Plan coordinated actions to meet needs and priorities by reviewing currently-used programmes/initiatives and, when needed, supplement with other evidence-based programmes • Identify success criteria for core team functioning, and measures of progress reflecting priorities, aims, and capacities based on programme logic within a specific context • Ensure ongoing resource allocation for professional development and learning, and implementation to maximise sustainability	• Involving key members of the school community in all implementation decisions maximises whole school commitment and ownership, which are essential foundations for change • Sharing data about readiness can facilitate an empowerment process and encourage participation • A structured approach documenting needs for change and identifying clear priorities and causal pathways helps keep the implementation and resource allocation focused and efficient, and thus provides a reference point for review • Building on existing effective programmes and approaches maximises positive outcomes and the efficient use of resources • Identifying intermediate outcomes to measure and celebrate progress and impact maintains motivation and ensures effective practice to achieve overall goal	Denman, 1999; McBride et al., 1999; Heward et al., 2007; Flaspohler et al., 2008; Elias et al., 2003; Kellogg Foundation, 2004; Green and Kreuter, 2005; Samdal et al., 2010; Weiner et al., 2008; Leurs et al., 2007; Dür 2012; Samdal, 2008; Firth et al., 2008; Inchley et al., 2007; Spillane, 2006; Leithwood et al., 2007; Hall and Hord, 2006

(Continued)

TABLE 5.1 (*Continued*)

How to implement the components	Why/rationale for how	Examples of literature for theoretical and empirical base
Policy and institutional anchoring		
• Build on existing policies and identify areas of strength and areas for action for school development	• Policy development and review provide a scaffold for school development	Bond et al., 2001; Hoyle et al., 2008; Samdal, 2008; Deschesnes et al., 2003;
• Identify concrete actions in the school policy plan, thereby documenting agreement of stakeholders to the plan and create readiness	• It can involve a vision, a mandate, decisions and actions, and a strategy for support	Daft, 1999; Samdal et al., 2010
• Stimulate alignment and commitment as a core implementation focus	• Policy facilitates institutional anchoring through specification of the provision of financial, organisational and technical resources	
Professional development (PD) and professional learning (PL)		
• Initial external PD of core team and executives for leadership	• Developing strategic and shared leadership and understanding through PD is critical to the change process	Boyd et al., 2006; Daft, 1999,Fullan, 1992, 2008; Tjomsland et al., 2009;
• Increase motivation and competence by school-based professional learning for whole staff	• PD and PL in priority areas is needed to build teacher efficacy for implementation and to maximise fidelity	Easton, 2008; Cole, 2008; Easton, 2008; Jourdan
• Embed PL in teachers' work	• External training provides an opportunity to build on experiences from other schools	2011; Mason and Rowling, 2005; Butler et al., 2011;
• External networking for executive staff and core team	• Internal PL develops a supportive context for school development and learning communities	Hall and Hord, 2006; Boot et al., 2010; Deschesnes
• Internal sharing of experiences and skill development through a range of PL strategies such as team building, mentoring and shadowing	• Coaching, skills training, competency building about development of trust for relationship building and reflective practice	et al., 2010; Rowling and Jeffreys, 2006; Jourdan, 2011; Butler et al., 2011;
• The presence of a 'critical friend' can facilitate school development	• Knowledge acquisition about educational change and innovation	Barnard et al., 2009
• Diverse and changing role expectations for external stakeholders necessitate professional learning opportunities		

Leadership and management practices

Actions	Rationale	References
• Anchor visions and aims in current school priorities • Use both leadership and management strategies • Share decision making, negotiate directions, understand change processes, build relationships • Identify a role model and provide opportunities for the staff to share and reflect on knowledge and experience, build leadership at many levels • Give feedback and acknowledge contribution • Monitor implementation and guide redirections when needed • Celebrate progress and achievements	• Leadership and management help to align visions and priorities stimulating commitment and fidelity to school community agreed actions • Role models and peer support increase teacher efficacy • Variety and complexity of tasks mean many leaders at different levels • Establishing a culture of reflective practice, feedback and acknowledgment of contribution enhances competence and stimulates commitment towards agreed actions • Monitoring implementation helps keep focus and provides basis for improvements	Spillane, 2006; Daft, 1999; Sabatier 1997; Samdal et al., 2010; Larsen and Samdal, 2008; Inchley et al., 2007; Center for Mental Health and Schools, 2006; Fullan, 1992, 2005; Rowling, 2009; Rowling and Mason, 2007; Larsen and Samdal, 2008

Relational and organisational support context

Actions	Rationale	References
• Integrate priority areas into written policies • Create caring environments in classrooms through pedagogic leadership • Modify and create appropriate physical spaces/buildings • Scaffold beneficial teaching schedules, class meetings, reflective behaviours and grouping to allow time and opportunities for collaboration and implementation • Focus on relationships as the foundation of pedagogy and student-centred learning • Build capacity by providing supportive ongoing conditions and physical and organisational structures for professional development and learning • Create eligibility for additional resources by linking with external agencies	• Policies represent the school's declaration of commitment • A supportive context can facilitate person-to-person and human–environment interactions beneficial to agreed aims • Time for collaboration is essential for school development • A positive climate enhances teaching, learning and thriving, and school connectedness • Relational pedagogy equips learners to become partners in their own learning • Processes are needed for sharing insights from PL	Larsen and Samdal, 2008; Durlak and Dupré, 2008; Aldinger et al., 2008; Samdal et al., 2010; Hall and Hord, 2006; MacNeill and Silcox, 2003; Boyd, et al., 2006; Cole, 2008; Jensen and Simovska, 2005; Samdal et al., 2010

(Continued)

TABLE 5.1 (*Continued*)

How to implement the components	Why/rationale for how	Examples of literature for theoretical and empirical base
Partnerships and networking • Invite parents to contribute to identifying school needs and to be represented in core team • Meetings and communication with relevant collaborators and, where appropriate, establish contracts including commitment and responsibilities • Develop partnerships requiring readiness, vision, leadership and time • Lateral capacity building through links with other schools by shadowing and exchange of staff for sharing and learning from each other	• Parents, as members of the core team, have an opportunity to share their expertise and ensure that the approach can be supported by the home setting • Sharing leadership and power increases participation and empowerment and prevents fragmentation • Regular information exchange and opportunities to contribute capitalise on the breadth of expertise of collaborators • Exposure to different models of implementation provides confirmation and opportunities of learning	Cuttance and Stokes 2000; Hoyle, 2008; Boot *et al.*, 2010; Heward *et al.*, 2007; Center for Mental Health and Schools, 2008; Deschesnes *et al.*, 2003; Deschesnes *et al.*, 2010; Samdal *et al.*, 2010; Clarke *et al.*, 2010 ; Fullan, 2005; Inchley *et al.*, 2007
Student participation • Student centred classroom with active decision making • Help young people learn that they can make a difference to self and others • Develop the ability in adults to put aside their views and trust in a young person's perspective and advice • Develop teacher skills to facilitate student participation • Create varying structures to facilitate students' influence and participation and invite them to be represented in core team • Ask and listen to students' perceptions of school needs for change and enable them to act on their ideas to address them in an inclusive and non-judgmental manner	• Formalising students' opportunities for school decision making establishes their involvement as a key operational mechanism and provides for the inclusion of their perspectives • Participation is increased using a developmental approach, increasing empowerment through sense of control, connectedness and meaning • Young people vary in their interests, skills and confidence and so different opportunities need to be available • Opportunities for voicing and acting on ideas helps to develop their competence and responsibility to act in a democratic society	Holdsworth and Blanchard, 2006; Jensen and Simovska, 2005; Leurs, *et al.*, 2007; Norman, 2001; Holdsworth and Blanchard, 2006; AICAFMHA, 2008; Simovska, 2008

Sustainability

- Review needs assessment and develop new priority areas
- Anchor initiative in written policies and learning outcomes
- Monitor and, where necessary, modify existing actions
- Continue with resource allocation
- PD and PL for new staff and provide booster sessions for existing staff
- Evaluate PL of staff, focusing on teacher and school administrator behaviour as indicators of system change

- Continuous follow-up and regular review help to maintain implementation efficiency and momentum
- Monitoring and reviewing identify the necessity for change in training needs, action, and/or resource allocation
- Steady and positive behaviour and organisational change ensures the majority of staff work towards agreed priorities

Fullan, 1992, 2001, 2005; Larsen and Samdal, 2008; Daft, 1999; Hazell *et al.*, 2002; Bond *et al.*, 2001; Sabatier, 1997; Inchley *et al.*, 2007; Firth *et al.*, 2008; Easton, 2008; Tjomsland *et al.*, 2009

Note

1 This chapter is based on the article by Rowling and Samdal, 2011: Filling the black box of implementation for health promoting schools. *Health Education*, 111(5), 347–366. © Emerald Publishing Group.

References

Aldinger, C., Zhang, X.-W., Liu, L.-Q., Guo, J.-X., Yu Sen Hai & Jones, J. (2008). Strategies for implementing Health-Promoting Schools in a province in China. *Promotion & Education*, *15*(1), 24–29.

Australian Infant Child Adolescent and Family Mental Health Association (2008). National Youth Participation Strategy Project Report, Commonwealth of Australia. Retrieved from http://www.aicafmha.net.au/youth_participation/index.html (accessed 21 September 2012).

Barnard, M., Becker, E., Creegan, C., Day, N., Devitt, K., Fuller, E., *et al.* (2009). *Evaluation of the National Healthy Schools Programme*. Interim Report. London: Department of Health.

Barry, M. M., Domitrovich, C. E. & Lara, M. A. (2005). The implementation of mental health promotion programme. *Promotion & Education*, *2*, 30–36.

Bond, L., Glover, S., Godfrey, C., Butler, H. & Patton, G. C. (2001). Building capacity for system-level change in schools: lessons from the gatehouse project. *Health Education & Behavior*, *28*(3), 368–383.

Boot, N., van Assama, P., Hesdal, B. & de Vries, N. (2010). Professional assistance in implementing school health policies. *Health Education*, *110*(4), 294–308.

Boyd, R., MacNeill, N. & Sullivan, G. (2006). Relational pedagogy: putting balance back into students' learning. *Curriculum Leadership*, *4*(13). www.curriculum.edu.au/leader/relational_pedagogy=putting_balance_back_into_stu,13944.html?issueID=10277 (accessed 25 September 2012).

Butler, H., Krelle, A., Seal, I., Trafford, L., Sarah, D., Hargreaves, J., *et al.* (2011). *The Critical Friend. Facilitating Change and Wellbeing in School Communities*. Camberwell: ACER Press.

Catford, J. (2009). Advancing the 'science of delivery' of health promotion: not just the 'science of discovery'. *Health Promotion International*, *24*(1), 1–5.

Center for Mental Health and Schools (2006). *Systemic Change and Empirically Supported Practices: The Implementation Problem*. Los Angeles, CA: Center for Mental Health and Schools.

Center for Mental Health and Schools. (2008). Working collaboratively: from school-based teams to school community higher education connections. Retrieved from http://smhp.psych.ucla.edu/pdfdocs/worktogether/worktogether.pdf (accessed 21 September 2012).

Clarke, A., O'Sullivan, M. & Barry, M. M. (2010). Context matters in programme implementation. *Health Education*, *110*(4), 273–293.

Cole, P. (2008). Inquiry into Effective Strategies for Professional Learning, V. Parliament (Ed.). Retrieved from http://www.parliament.vic.gov.au/etc/Submissions/prof_learn/cole270308.pdf (accessed 12 April 2012).

Cuttance, P. & Stokes, S. (2000). Reporting on Student and School Achievement. A Research Report prepared for the Commonwealth Department of Education, Training and Youth Affairs.. Canberra. Retrieved from http://www.dest.gov.au/

sectors/school_education/publications_resources/other_publications/reporting_on_
student_and_school_achievement.htm (accessed 12 April 2012).

Daft, R. L. (1999). *Leadership: Theory and Practice*. Fort Worth, TX: Dryden Press.

Denman, S. (1999). Health promoting schools in England – a way forward in development. *Journal of Public Health Medicine, 21*(2), 215–220.

Deschesnes, M., Martin, C. & Hill, A. J. (2010). Comprehensive approaches to school
health promotion: how to achieve broader implementation? *Health Promotion
International, 18*(4), 387–396.

Dusenbury, L., Brannigan, R., Falco, M. & Hansen, W. B. (2003). A review of research
on fidelity of implementation: implications for drug abuse prevention in school
settings. *Health Education Research, 18*(2), 237–256.

Easton, L. B. (2008). From professional development to professional learning. *Phi Delta
Kappa, 89*(10), 755–759.

Elias, M. J., Zins, J., Graczyk, P. & Weissberg, R. (2003). Implementation, sustainability,
and scaling up of social-emotional and academic innovations in public schools. *School
Psychology Review 32*, 303–319.

Firth, N., Butler, H., Drew, S., Krell, A., Sheffield, J., Patton, G. C., *et al.* (2008).
Implementing multilevel programs and approaches that address student wellbeing and
connectedness: Factoring in the needs of the school. *Advances in School Mental Health
Promotion, 1*(4), 14–24.

Flaspohler, P., Duffy, J., Wandersman, A., Stillman, L. & Maras, M. (2008).
Unpacking prevention capacity: an intersection of research-to-practice models
and community-centered models. *American Journal of Community Psychology, 41*(3),
182–196.

Fullan, M. (1992). *Successful School Improvement*. Toronto, Canada: OISE Press.

Fullan, M. (2005a, b). *Leadership and Sustainability. System Thinkers in Action*. Thousand
Oaks, CA: Corwin Press.

Fullan, M. (2008). *The Six Secrets of Change. What the Best Leaders Do to Help Their
Organizations Survive and Thrive*. San Fransisco, CA: Jossey-Bass.

Green, L. W. & Kreuter, M. W. (2005). *Health Programme Planning: An Educational and
Ecological Approach* (4th edn). New York, NY: McGraw-Hill.

Hargreaves, A., Earl, L., Moore, S. & Manning, S. (2001). *Learning to Change. Teaching
Beyond Subjects and Standards*. San Francisco, CA: Jossey-Bass Inc.

Hazell, T., Vincent, K., Waring, T. & Lewin, T. (2002). The challenges of
evaluating national mental health promotion programs in schools: A case study using
the evaluation of MindMatters. *International Journal of Mental Health Promotion, 4*(4),
21–27.

Heward, S., Hutchins, C. & Keleher, H. (2007). Organizational change – key to
capacity building and effective health promotion. *Health Promotion International, 22*(2),
170–178.

Holdsworth, R. & Blanchard, M. (2006). Unheard voices: themes emerging from studies
of the views about school engagement of young people with high support needs in the
area of mental health. *Australian Journal of Guidance and Counselling, 16*(1), 14–28.

Hoyle, T. B., Samek, B. B. & Valois, R. F. (2008). Building capacity for the continuous
improvement of health-promoting schools. *Journal of School Health, 78*(1), 1–8.

Inchley, J., Muldoon, J. & Currie, C. (2007). Becoming a health promoting school:
evaluating the process of effective implementation in Scotland. *Health Promotion
International, 22*(1), 65–71. d

Jensen, B. B. & Simovska, V. (2005). Involving students in learning and health promotion
processes – clarifying what? how? and why? *Promotion & Education, 12*(3–4), 150–156.

Jonnaert, P., Barrette, J. & Masciotra, D. (2006). Revising the Concept of Competence as an Organizing Principle for Programs of Study: From Competence to Competent Action. Retrieved from http://www.ibe.unesco.org (accessed 12 April 2012).

Jourdan, D. (2011). *Health Education in Schools. The Challenges of Teacher Training.* Saint-Denis: INPES.

Kellogg Foundation. (2004). Logic Model Development Guide. Retrieved from http://www.wkkf.org (accessed 21 September 2012).

Larsen, T. & Samdal, O. (2008). Facilitating the implementation and sustainability of second step. *Scandinavian Journal of Educational Research, 52*(2), 187–204.

Leeder, S. R. (1997). Health-promoting environments: the role of public policy. *Australian and New Zealand Journal of Public Health, 21*(4), 413–414.

Leurs, M. T. W., Bessems, K., Schaalma, H. P. & de Vries, H. (2007). Focus points for school health promotion improvements in Dutch primary schools. *Health Education Research, 22*(1), 58–69.

Lister-Sharp, D., Chapman, S., Stewart-Brown, S. & Sowden, A. (1999). Health promoting schools and health promotion in school: two systematic reviews. *Health Technology Assessment 3*(22), 1–207.

Lowry-Webster, H.M., Barrett, P.M. & Lock, S. (2003). A universal prevention trial of anxiety symptomology during childhood: Results at one-year follow-up. *Behaviour Change,* 20(1), 25–43.

Mason, J. & Rowling, L. (2005). Look after the staff first – a case study of developing staff health and well-being. *Promotion and Education, 12*(3–4), 140.

Norman, J. (2001). Building effective youth-adult partnerships. *Transitions, 14*(1), 10–12.

Olweus, D. (1993). *Bullying at School: What We Know and What We Can Do.* Oxford: Blackwell Publishers.

Patton, M. (2004). *Utilization-Focused Evaluation* (3rd edn). Thousand Oaks, CA: Sage Publications.

Rowling, L. (2008). Prevention science and implementation of school mental health promotion and prevention and wellbeing: another way. *Advances in School Mental Health Promotion, 1*(3), 29–37.

Rowling, L. (2009). Strengthening "school" in school mental health promotion. *Health Education, 109*(4), 357–368.

Rowling, L. & Mason, J. (2005). A case study of multi-method evaluation of complex school mental health promotion and prevention: the MindMatters evaluation suite. *Australian Journal of Guidance and Counselling, 15*(2), 125–136.

Rowling, L. & Samdal, O. (2011). Filling the black box of implementation for health-promoting schools. *Health Education, 111*(5), 347–366.

Sabatier, P. A. (1997). Top-down and bottom-up approaches to implementation research. In M. Hill (Ed.), *The Policy Process: A Reader* (2nd edn, pp. 272–295) Harlow: Pearson/Harvester Wheatsheaf.

Samdal, O. (2008). School health promotion. In H. Heggenhougen (Ed.), *The Encyclopedia of Public Health* (Vol. 5, pp. 653–661). Oxford: Elsevier Inc.

Samdal, O. & Rowling, L. (2011). Theoretical and empirical base for implementation components of health promoting schools. *Health Education, 3*(5), 367–390.

Samdal, O., Viig, N. G. & Wold, B. (2010). Health promotion integrated into school policy and practice: experiences of implementation in the Norwegian network of health promoting schools. *Journal of Child and Adolescent Psychology, 1*(2), 43–72.

Scottish Health Promoting Schools Unit. (2004). Being Well – Doing Well. A framework for health promoting schools in Scotland. Retrieved from http://www. ltscotland.org.uk/Images/Beingwelldoingwell_tcm4-121991.pdf (accessed 12 April 2012).

Simovska, V. (2008), Learning in and as participation. In Reid, A., Jensen, B.B., Nikel, J. and Simovska, V. (Eds), *Participation and Learning. Perspectives in Education and Environment, Health and Sustainability.* New York: Springer, pp. 61–80.

Spillane, J. (2006). *Distributed Leadership.* San Francisco, CA: Jossey-Bass.

Stewart-Brown, S. (2006). What is the evidence on school health promotion in improving health or preventing disease and, specifically, what is the effectiveness of the health promoting schools approach? *Health Evidence Network Report.* Copenhagen: WHO Regional Office for Europe.

Tjomsland, H. E., Iversen, A. C. & Wold, B. (2009). The Norwegian network of health promoting schools: a three-year follow-up study of teacher motivation, participation and perceived outcomes. *Scandinavian Journal of Educational Research, 53*(1), 89–102.

Weiner, B. J., Lewis, M. A. & Linnan, L. A. (2009). Using organization theory to understand the determinants of effective implementation of worksite health promotion programs. *Health Education Research, 24*(2), 292–305.

Whitelaw, S., Martin, C., Kerr, A. & Wimbush, E. (2006). An evaluation of the Health Promoting Health Service Framework: the implementation of a settings based approach within the NHS in Scotland. *Health Promotion International, 21*(2), 136–144.

PART II

Case studies[1]

The next four chapters provide concrete examples of implementation approaches in different regions and countries. Each case study highlights how the specific country's context influenced implementation at school level and exemplifies how some of the components operated within this context. These factors include socio-cultural components, geopolitical aspects, resources, and diverse educational and health systems.

Note

1   Recommended citation for case studies: case study author(s) (2013); case study title. Chapter #, chapter title. In O. Samdal and L. Rowling (Eds), *Implementation of Health Promoting Schools: Explaining the theories of what, why and how* (pp. xx–xx). London: Routledge.

6

CANADA AND NORWAY

Leadership and management at regional and school level

As highlighted in Chapters 4 and 5, clear leadership in building school ownership and capacity are key strategies for successful implementation of health promotion in schools. At school level the key person in building owner-ship of the health promoting organisational change process is the principal in that he or she is in a core position to motivate the stakeholders (students, staff, parents and collaborators) to carry out the needed actions. Further, the principal and school leadership can prioritise resources and time to stimulate a supportive context for the implementation. Leadership is, however, not only important at school level. Clear leadership at regional and national level giving priority and support to implementation of health promotion at school level represents a crit-ical source for stimulating concrete actions at school level. The two case studies in this chapter from Canada and Norway demonstrate the importance of these two leadership levels.

The case study from the province of Alberta in Canada provides a view of policy and practice development in an educational division. The appointment of a health facilitator to guide the work, the growth in this position to a senior administrative position on the educational leadership team, with responsibility for the Collaborative Initiatives and Partnerships Department, anchored the activity within both the education and health systems. This was supported by multiple governmental, regional and community partnerships. Curriculum developments at a provincial level enhanced the work at the divisional level. The systemic leadership approach at provincial level provided a foundation that was sustained despite organisational changes and clearly stimulated school-based initiatives.

The importance of strong leadership at school level emerged as a key area of the health promoting schools initiative in Norway over a 10-year period. Two components, visionary leadership, and management of resources built the capacity of staff, motivating them through democratic processes, such as all staff agreeing to take up the health promoting schools policy. Such processes also contributed to the development of staff shared values, readiness for change and ownership of action. The existing education environment focus on test scores for numeracy and literacy threatened the health promotion vision, necessitating that school leaders maintained their commitment and continued to emphasise the contribution of health promoting schools to learning. Along with the vision and commitment, management of resources relating to the school's professional learning and daily routines needed to sustain a focus on health. Effective resource management and a collaborative culture, contributed to motivation and whole school ownership.

EDUCATION AND HEALTH SECTOR ORGANISATIONAL CHANGE FOR SCHOOL HEALTH DEVELOPMENT IN CANADA

Gloria Wells

The setting for this case study is the division-wide, integrated approach to the development of school-based health, mental health, family support, and mentoring initiatives within Rocky View School Division, an urban/rural school division serving 34 schools and 16,000 students in southern Alberta, Canada, from 1996 to 2010.

The two components of implementation, *Policy and institutional anchoring*, and *Leadership and management practices* will be elaborated in this case study. The context required that the Policy and institutional anchoring be systemic within both the education and health sectors seeking to implement effective school based health initiatives. In addition, it was critical that they were cross-systemic in conceptualisation, implementation support, and accountability for outcomes achieved. Both policy and institutional anchoring became integrated, and articulated as such, within the broader mandates of both organisations, as well as understood to be the foundational prerequisite for the joint efforts represented through the School Health initiatives undertaken.

Context

Throughout the 14 years of development described in this case study, there were a number of contextual factors that must be noted.

1. At the outset, beginning in 1995, the Calgary Health Region, which served the Rocky View School Division, as well as the two major Calgary school boards, initiated Comprehensive School Health programming in schools by funding an embedded School Health Facilitator, an education specialist with knowledge and interest in health promotion selected by the school jurisdiction for a three-year period. This was a critical support to school

jurisdictions, whose provincial funding from the Education Ministry was limited to providing for direct educational costs.

2. Within Rocky View School Division, this position evolved over the years to become a senior administrative position within the divisional educational leadership team, which oversaw the Collaborative Initiatives and Partnerships Department, fully integrated into the mandate, educational planning and programming undertaken on behalf of the jurisdiction. This evolution was unique to this school division and laid the path to the development and implementation of coordinated programming for all schools in the division of a wide range of health, mental health and other programmes across the service continuum. These were under the auspices of the Rocky View Schools Health Promoting Schools Framework, and funded through multiple governmental, regional and community partners, including a number of initiatives aimed at supporting school staff. The School Health Facilitator position ended in 2010 due to staff changes, and other functions of the department being diversified throughout the division's infrastructure.

3. From the outset, all school jurisdictions involved and the Calgary Health Region formed a Comprehensive School Health Steering Group, which assisted collaboration and joint problem solving around systemic requirements and issues involved in this regional implementation. The regional Calgary Rocky View Health Promoting Schools Collaborative is still in existence, continuing to provide support. Links to Alberta Wellness, the Health Ministry for Alberta, evolved as well over the years from being primarily an arms-length funder to the Calgary Health Region for Health Promotion initiatives, to an active participant in regional activity via involved staff under the centralised Alberta Health Services, which under ministerial order, combined all nine provincial health jurisdictions. This has led to more cross-systems collaboration at the provincial level with a cross-ministry School Health Manager, as well as membership in the Pan Canadian Consortium for School Health, with representatives from all provincial ministries except Quebec.

4. Provincial initiatives in Education facilitated this work. The development of a new K–12 curriculum, implemented from 2012, has provided some impetus for school districts to incorporate a 'comprehensive school health' approach. As well, an Alberta cross-ministry 'Healthy Kids' mandate leading to a provincial school nutrition strategy and enhanced physical activity initiatives, along with the appointment of six regional School Health Facilitators, has continued to provide a broad basis of support for comprehensive school health initiatives provincially. Incongruently, there is currently very limited funding, either through Education or Health funding streams, to school jurisdictions to implement desired health promotion programmes, even though provincial school based educational accountability measures now include some indicators relating directly to Comprehensive School Health implementation.

Systemic and organisationally integrated policy development and institutional anchoring

The foundational principles underpinning the policies related to collaborative and integrative approaches undertaken to maximise the levels of collaboration and partnering in Rocky View Schools, were adopted from a seminal document by Franklin and Streeter (1995), which sought to identify a number of implementation factors with various approaches to linking schools and human services. They identified the approaches as: Informal Relations, Coordination, Partnership, Collaboration and Integration. The components they identified to be developed within each approach are: Commitment, Planning, Training, Leadership Patterns, Resources, Funding, Scope of Change, and Impact.

The Health Promoting Schools Framework (Wells, Bandali & Maloff, 2009) provided the operational framework for the design and development of all health-related initiatives implemented during this time. Subsequently it was applied to a Healthy Eating Initiative (2007–2010), figure 6.1. The collaboration with, and integral involvement of, contributing partners, including participating schools, was predicated upon their understanding of, and agreement with, the inclusion of all the components described therein, to the design and implementation of initiatives and programmes.

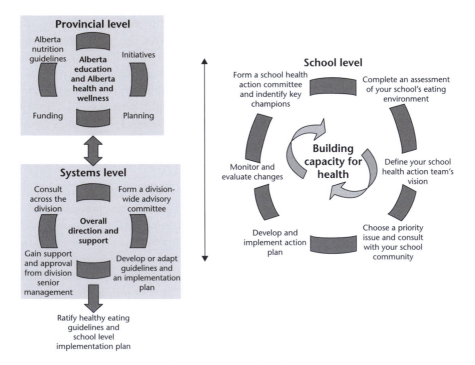

FIGURE 6.1 The overview of framework for school improvement

Source: Wells, Bandali & Maloff (2009)

Institutional anchoring was accomplished by the presence of the Collaborative Initiatives Department and its director on the divisional leadership team, the incorporation of a goal and outcome into the school division's three year plan tied specifically to the efforts of the range of initiatives unified under the auspices of 'addressing non-academic barriers to learning'. By affirming that these barriers can impede a student's ability to learn (University of Miami at Ohio), it became viable to link health and mental health related programming directly to learning outcomes (Rocky View Schools Plan 2008–2011), which can facilitate their integration into all of the work of the jurisdiction within the context of school improvement, as was done by this author through the schema represented in Figure 6.1, the 'Overview of Framework for School Improvement' (Wells, Bandali & Maloff, 2009).

Congruent health and education sector leadership and management practices

Leadership and management practices that both facilitated and modelled the specific attributes of collaboration and integration defined by the Franklin Streeter Schema (1995) and that maximised the outcomes experienced include the following components:

- Presence of credible educational administrator within the school jurisdictional leadership team with capacity to work effectively within the educational mandate while having credibility in the health sector to facilitate collaboration and partnership with senior level health and human service infrastructures.
- Development of regional infrastructure (Calgary Rocky View Health Promoting Collaborative) to facilitate senior administrative level, cross-sectoral planning and problem solving.
- Development of a school jurisdictional infrastructure (Rocky View Schools Health Promoting Schools Advisory Council), to be an inclusive, representative body (principals, teachers, support staff, students, community allied professionals), to engage input for appropriate implementation directions and strategies, link to school-based action groups, as well as build capacity in members regarding Health Promoting Schools' principles and models.
- Cross organisation agreements regarding resource sharing, joint supervision (e.g. the health sector providing money for health or education, staff located within the school jurisdiction), and joint evaluation/accountability mechanisms.
- Conceptualisation of mechanisms that will facilitate information sharing and organisational support at all levels.

Outcomes

Some indicators that this approach was successful include:

1. By 2008, school health and health programming in general was incorporated in the jurisdictional strategic plan, with identified outcomes and indicators.
2. By 2009, 100% of schools in the division had school health related goals in their individual School Education Plans.
3. By 2008, 100% of schools had adopted the Rocky View Nutritional Guidelines and incorporated school nutrition goals in their annual School Education Plan.
4. In 2008, Rocky View Schools, the Calgary Region of Alberta Health Services and Devon Energy received the Mayors' Excellence Award for Outstanding School Based Education and Health Partnership.

It was necessary that specific Leadership and management practices were identified and facilitated in both systems to ensure congruency, within and across, in order to maximise organisational direction and support to benefit regional and school based staff from organisations, students, parents and community-based partners.

From 1996–2010, The Collaborative Initiatives Department was home to approximately 30 various health, mental health and human services staff, all supported through partnerships, supporting the health and well-being of 16,000 students through school based health and human services initiatives, across the continuum of programming from universal, comprehensive approaches to targeted service initiatives. While the department was discontinued in 2010, a foundation was laid that provided for a number of the school-based initiatives to continue on within the context of an overarching goal of the division to attend to the reduction of barriers to learning, and individual school plans to incorporate health related strategies into their annual plans.

FROM INITIATION TO INSTITUTIONALISATION: THE PRINCIPALS' LEADERSHIP AND MANAGEMENT IN NORWEGIAN HEALTH PROMOTING SCHOOLS

Hege Eikeland Tjomsland, Oddrun Samdal, Nina Grieg Viig and Bente Wold

Introduction

This case study focuses on the experiences of 10 Norwegian Health Promoting Schools (HPS) during enrolment in the European Network of HPS from 1993 to 2003. It looks specifically at how the school leaders worked to ensure that the HPS policy was implemented and sustained in school over time. The key components concerning school leadership referred to in this case study have been identified through previous studies from the Norwegian network.

The Norwegian context

In Norwegian elementary and junior high schools, the leader group usually consists of a principal and one to three school department leaders and counsellors depending on the school size. In the following, *school leader* will refer to an employee in the leader group.

The Norwegian HPS project management provided few guidelines concerning the leaders' involvement in the HPS, although it was emphasised that the school leaders ought to actively support the implementation of the HPS policy. This was also highlighted in a two-day seminar focusing on health promotion offered to all the school leaders and one additional teacher in each school at the onset of the network period.

The evaluation of the Norwegian HPS showed that the HPS policy was more easily implemented in schools where the leaders worked side by side with teachers to lead as well as manage (Tjomsland, Larsen, Viig & Wold, 2009). Here, the HPS was granted status even if the school leaders did not participate at an operational level in health promotion. After ten years, schools with leaders who had exerted visionary leadership in health promotion as well as management mobilising resources for health promotion, had been the most successful in integrating the HPS policy into the daily fabric of school life (Samdal, Viig & Wold, 2010; Tjomsland, Larsen, Samdal & Wold, 2010). In the following, a more detailed account from the Norwegian studies demonstrates how the school leaders led as well as managed their HPS.

The visionary leader

First, the evaluation of the Norwegian HPS indicates that staff perceived the school leader as an important motivating agent for the HPS (Tjomsland *et al.*, 2010). In schools where the school leaders felt responsible for and actually set aside time to motivate staff for health promotion, the teachers were more eager and willing to implement the HPS policy than in other schools. A case study in one of the HPS applying mixed methods found, for example, that the school leaders' ability to establish commitment in the staff contributed to a sustained and extended physical activity practice during the 10-year study period (Tjomsland, Larsen, Samdal & Wold, 2010). The findings from surveys among teachers at baseline and at three year follow-up (n=104) further suggested that the school leaders' support of the HPS policy was regarded by the teachers as an important condition enabling their participation (Viig, Tjomsland & Wold, 2010). The most efficient school leaders motivated staff through a democratic process in which all teachers agreed to take up a HPS policy. And even if the school leaders signalled strong personal commitment to the HPS policy and knew where they wanted the school to be headed, they facilitated discussions in staff allowing them to share contradicting beliefs and attitudes. In this way, they enabled joint reflections about the positive outcomes of school health promotion contributing to a set of shared values and readiness for change among the staff.

Second, it was crucial that the school leaders did not lose interest in health promotion, but held on to and reinforced visions and aspirations in health promotion during times of change (Tjomsland, Larsen *et al.*, 2009). Like schools in other European countries, Norwegian schools have been under immense pressure to improve test scores in literacy and numeracy during the past decade. In an increasingly market oriented school political climate, teachers may easily push health promotion issues to a peripheral position if they are not supported by school leaders with a strong commitment to the HPS (Tjomsland *et al.*, 2009). It was therefore essential that the school leaders held on to and communicated to staff that the HPS policy contributed positively to their teaching and learning programme.

In addition to being committed to the HPS, the most notable school leaders kept abreast of school political discussions and developments in health promotion (Tjomsland *et al.*, 2010). For example, a national policy recommendation encouraging schools to promote daily physical activity at the beginning of this century was singled out early and actions undertaken. Interestingly, these schools became some of the pioneers in how to enable daily physical activity in school, and some of them were appointed by the government as model schools for physical activity promotion.

Finally, some school leaders deliberately linked the HPS to the ongoing life of the school as well as to the national curriculum when introducing the HPS policy to staff (Viig, Fosse, Samdal & Wold, 2011). By using the teachers' daily practice and the school's current priorities as the starting point for the development of a more explicit and pronounced health promoting practice, the chance of integration and sustainability of the HPS improved. The teachers in these schools reported that such a strategy created positive attitudes and commitment in staff because it was not something new, an additional burden, which came on top of what they were already doing.

The manager

Although commitment and shared visions of health promotion among the staff served as a cornerstone for the implementation of the HPS policy, evaluation of the Norwegian HPS indicated that visionary leadership was combined with management enabling the teachers to get involved in health promotion (Samdal *et al.*, 2010; Tjomsland *et al.*, 2009; Viig *et al.*, 2011).

First, a formalisation of the HPS policy into plans and curriculum was a key strategy for its implementation and sustainability (Viig & Wold, 2005). Once the HPS policy had been written into the schools' plans and curricula, the teachers were more committed because they could not ignore a priority area (Samdal et al., 2010). Moreover, the formalisation of the HPS into school documents stimulated the transfer of experience and made staff less dependent on teachers with special interests and qualifications in health promotion (Viig et al., 2011).

Second, it proved efficient also after the initiation, to earmark time for discussions and critical reflections among the staff related to how they were doing and where they wanted to go in terms of health promotion (Viig et al., 2011). One school even set aside one student-free day at the beginning of each school year to introduce the school's pedagogical platform and health promotion practices to new teachers. Through systematic use of evaluation the school leaders ensured constant renewal in health promotion and opportunities for staff to develop and improve. As such the school leaders also mitigated teachers' loss of interest in the field and the abandonment of established practices.

Third, the case study from one of the HPS indicates that the opportunity for all teachers to participate in training in health promotion contributed positively to the integration of physical activity into the schools' daily operations (Tjomsland et al., 2010). By providing training opportunities also for teachers who were not eager to get involved, the school leaders ensured that feelings of ownership for the HPS were created among all members of staff rather than only among teachers with a personal interest and competence in health promotion. It was, however, important that the school leaders were aware of the teachers' different strengths and weaknesses and allowed for alternative responsibilities and assignments.

A fourth notable characteristic of a particularly efficient HPS, was a teacher climate characterised by collaboration among the teachers in terms of sharing ideas and methods as well as responsibilities and challenges in health promotion (Tjomsland et al., 2010; Viig et al., 2010). Collaboration between teachers was possible because the school leaders created timetables and teaching schedules allowing for an exchange of experience. As such, it was possible for staff to share responsibilities in health promotion and further to take advantage of teachers' different competencies in health promotion. Not surprisingly, schools that emphasised collaboration reported higher integration of health promotion practices into the daily fabric of the teachers' professional lives than schools without the same emphasis on collaboration in health promotion.

Finally, the teachers' motivation to be engaged increased through collaboration with external partners (Tjomsland, Wold & Iversen, 2009). In particular, networking with other HPS yielded ample opportunities for improved teacher collaboration and professional learning (Viig et al., 2011). Both interview data and survey data at three year follow-up, suggested that networking both within school and with other HPS in Norway and abroad was highly associated with teachers' participation in health promotion (Viig, Tjomsland & Wold, 2010; Viig & Wold, 2005). Collaboration with other HPS may have been particularly attractive and stimulating for the school leaders who pointed to increased competence in how to lead development and implementation processes in schools through national and international networking (Viig *et al.*, 2011).

Reflections and lessons learned

Studies from the Norwegian HPS suggest that school leaders in charge of implementing and sustaining the HPS policy ought to exert both visionary leadership and management. Visionary leadership refers to how the school leaders set the tone for the implementation of the HPS policy and fostered a climate in staff that responded positively to the HPS policy during times of change. Management, on the other hand, refers to how the school leaders translated the HPS policy into practice through a formalisation of the policy into plans and curricula as well as through the creation of structures that supported productive working relations in health promotion. Equally important was the opportunity for staff to participate in professional training in health promotion.

Even if the Norwegian HPS network never reached widespread dissemination, the HPS policy has been integrated into the two most recent school reforms (1997, 2006). Likewise, several White Papers and Propositions from the past decade point to health promotion as a vital aspect in the daily fabric of school life.

References

Franklin, C. & Streeter, C. (1995). School reform: linking public schools with human services. *Social Work*, *40*(6), 773–782.

Rocky View Schools Plan 2008–2011 from http://www.rocky view.ab.ca/publications/assets_publications/threeyearplans/threeyearplan20082011.pdf (accessed September 2008).

Samdal, O., Viig, N. G. & Wold, B. (2010). Health promotion integrated into school policy and practice: experiences of implementation in the Norwegian network of health promoting schools. *Journal of Child and Adolescent Psychology*, *2*, 43–72.

Tjomsland, H. E., Larsen, T., Samdal, O. & Wold, B. (2010). Sustaining comprehensive physical activity practice in elementary school: A case study applying mixed methods. *Teachers and Teaching: Theory and Practice*, *16*(1), 73–95.

Tjomsland, H. E., Larsen, T. B., Viig, N. G. & Wold, B. (2009). A fourteen year follow-up study of health promoting schools in Norway: principals' perceptions of conditions influencing sustainability. *The Open Education Journal*, *2*, 54–64.

Tjomsland, H. E., Wold, B. & Iversen, A. C. (2009). The Norwegian network of health promoting schools: a three-year follow-up study of teacher motivation, participation and perceived outcomes. *Scandinavian Journal of Educational Research*, *53*(10, 89–102.

University of Miami at Ohio (2007). Ohio Mental Health Network for Success in Schools. Information Brief: Non-Academic Barriers to Learning, from http://www.units.muohio.edu/csbmhp/network/barriers.pdf (accessed August 2007).

Viig, N. G., Fosse, E., Samdal, O. & Wold, B. (2011). Leading and supporting the implementation of the Health promoting schools program in Norway. *Scandinavian Journal of Educational Research*, 1–14.

Viig, N. G., Tjomsland, H. E. & Wold, B. (2010). Program and school characteristics related to teacher participation in school health promotion. *The Open Education Journal*, *3–11*(10–20).

Viig, N. G. & Wold, B. (2005). Facilitating teachers' participation in school-based health promotion – a qualitative study. *Scandinavian Journal of Educational Research*, *49*(1), 83–109.

Wells, G., Bandali, F., and Maloff, B. (2009). Rocky View School Division Collaborative Initiatives Department Planning. (Unpublished).

7

ENGLAND AND AUSTRALIA

Policy and institutional anchoring at national and regional level and its importance for sustainability

Within the implementation components of policy and institutional anchoring, organisational support context, and sustainability, there is a focus on the need to build a country and regional scaffold to enclose and support school level implementation. Such a formal framework delineates the parameters within which action can occur, be monitored and reviewed. Change within this structure, such as in government priorities, can support or weaken implementation. Issues such as resources, leadership at various levels, consultative processes, the climate and culture and technical capacity are elements within these components. Case studies from England and Australia illustrate these elements.

England developed a strong policy structure in both the health and education sectors. The National Healthy School Standard represented the political desire for 'joined up' action. Implementation leadership to assist schools to meet the standards' criteria occurred at Local Education Authority and Primary Care Trust levels with the support of other agencies. These partnerships were assisted by the National Healthy Schools programme. Organisational support and leadership was given by an across government Programme Board, existing advocacy groups and the Office for Standards in Education (Ofsted). The political priority of the focus on the 'whole child' also supported action. Withdrawal of funding at a national level, in part due to the global financial crisis in 2011, diminished activity due to loss of grants at local level. However, in the Leeds area, where there was early and continued support of the Primary Health Trust and a strong leader from health, the work is ongoing. Equally, the concept is actively sustained where schools have used it to promote pupil well-being and learning.

In Australia, the policy development occurred at state level, with national government funding the Australian Health Promoting Schools Association (AHPSA), to conduct benchmarking research and consult within the states and territories, to develop a national strategy. This national context of different state jurisdictions with responsibility for health and education resulted in varying documents but the desired outcomes for schools were similar. The leadership comes from state level and through the major national networking vehicle of the AHPSA. Funding comes from state based initiatives and, as in England, the concept has been absorbed into new national projects. The dynamic nature of health promoting schools and shifting health priorities results in organisations like AHPSA needing to modify their ways of networking and building capacity.

THE ENGLISH NATIONAL HEALTHY SCHOOLS PROGRAMME 1999–2011

Colin Noble and Marilyn Toft

Introduction

A series of policy initiatives in England created a relational and organisational environment where addressing health through schools was a key policy focus in government departments and local authorities. This case study focuses on these initiatives, their political context and its implication for sustainability.

Policy and institutional anchoring

In England the National Healthy School Standard (later known as the National Healthy Schools Programme) was launched in October 1999. It was an expression of the newly elected (1997) Labour Government's commitment to addressing the obvious gaps in health and education between the social classes. The rationale for the launch of the Standard was based on a number of reports that had been written in previous years, e.g. 'The Black Report' (Black, 1980), demonstrating that although overall health had improved since the introduction of the welfare state, there were widespread health inequalities. The main cause of these inequalities was economic inequality. The second report, commissioned by the Labour Government in 1997, aimed to examine health inequalities. This report 'Independent Inquiry into Inequalities in Health' (Acheson, 1998), largely echoed the earlier Black Report. The 1999 Department of Health White Paper, 'Saving Lives: Our Healthier Nation' and the Education White Paper of 1997, 'Excellence in Schools' committed the government to introduce a national healthy school standard.

From the outset the National Healthy School Standard was different from previous interventions. It was an expression of the new regime's determination to achieve 'joined up government' – a very popular aspiration in the late 1990s and early 2000s – and so was controlled and directed by both the Department of Health and the Department of Education. In many ways this was a novelty as very few programmes had two sponsoring departments. It was hosted and managed by the relatively new Health Development Agency, which was a 'quango' (quasi-autonomous non-governmental organisation) of the Department of Health.

At the beginning it was realised that if the Standard were to be successful it would have to be led and managed locally as well as nationally. In England there was a strong tradition of schools looking to their local education authorities (LEAs), locally elected councils, for such leadership and management. The Health Service had just established local primary care groups (later, Primary Care Trusts or 'PCTs') to run local health services, including health promotion schemes. So, the synergistic national partnership between the Departments of Education and Health was mirrored locally by partnerships between LEAs and PCTs.

Relational and organisational support context

Other government bodies and authorities such as Government Offices of the Regions, local healthy school partnerships and national healthy schools teams in the Health Development Agency, supported schools to meet a number of criteria around their capacity, competence and sustainability to achieve requirements of the national healthy school standard. The national government set a target that all 150 local healthy school programmes had to meet the criteria by 2002. While it provided annual grant to local councils (mostly used to employ local healthy schools coordinators), it did not make the programme compulsory for either LEAs or schools.

Nationally, the programme was supported by the establishment of a Programme Board with representatives of Health and Education and many other government departments including Transport, Food Standards, Culture, Media and Sport, and the Home Office (drugs) – all of whom had an interest in the success of the programme. Although the Programme Board experienced frustration, as there was generally very little understanding of how schools actually worked, the existence of such a large and influential group of stakeholders was undoubtedly a strength of the programme.

National support was also found in building relationships with existing advocacy groups and sympathetic organisations such as the National Health Education Group and the National Standing Conference of advisers, inspectors and consultants in Personal and Social Education, both of which had been in existence since the 1980s and had a great deal of influence in professional journals and LEAs. Another critical national relationship was with the Office for Standards in Education (Ofsted) – the schools' inspection agency. Ofsted, whose inspections of schools became both feared and authoritative in equal measure, was originally interested in the National Healthy Schools Programme because of the impact it might have on the academic standards attained by pupils. However, following the introduction of *Every Child Matters* in 2003 and the subsequent Education Act of 2004, schools were expected to support the development of children based on five outcomes:

1. being healthy;
2. staying safe;
3. enjoying and achieving;
4. making a positive contribution;
5. economic well-being.

This both greatly broadened the school's remit and, at the same time, made the National Healthy Schools Programme relevant to all schools. In reality, schools still put far more stress on the 'achieving' outcome than the others, as did Ofsted, but there was at least a token acknowledgement of the development of the 'whole child'. It forced a philosophical reflection about the contribution the other outcomes might make to pupil achievement.

Partnership and networking

The environment of support described above stresses the importance of partnership to the National Healthy School Programme. It became increasingly obvious that the vast majority of societal issues – and the programmes that were initiated – were complex and interconnected, incapable of being addressed effectively by one specialist agency. The National Healthy School Standard/ Programme, with its focus on the whole child and its insistence on a 'whole-school approach', depended more than most on partnership working and networking. Thus, regional networks of local healthy school coordinators were established based on the nine regional government offices. Meetings were held in which local experience and expertise could be shared between localities, messages from the national team given and debated, and regional speakers invited to present.

Sustainability

The National Healthy Schools Programme was always a highly political programme, in the sense that it had to bend and sway to satisfy developing government policy and meet the wishes of ministers. For example, the national and political concerns expressed about childhood obesity in 2005–6 resulted in greater emphasis being placed by the Programme on healthy eating and physical activity. The Coalition Government (Conservatives and Liberal Democrats) withdrew the funding from the Programme in April 2011. The national team disappeared overnight and local councils, already affected by heavy financial cuts, lost their grants. In many areas the local healthy schools team has been disbanded. In other areas, e.g. Leeds, the continuing programme is now called Healthy Schools and Well-Being rather than Healthy Schools. The Leeds programme has been sustained due to early and continued support of the local

Primary Care Trust with strong leadership from a figure in public health, and subsequently, the local council. Early decisions that contributed to sustainability were to invest heavily in health-related data and reporting capacity; to become a 'traded service' i.e. charging schools via agreements for their services; the maintenance of a large team able to offer a wide breadth of expertise and professional development; and the quality of the team together with its management and leadership.

However, in many schools a different sort of sustainability has occurred, one where schools have sustained the healthy schools approach by promoting pupil well-being as a means of helping pupils to achieve i.e. they have invested in pupil care, guidance and support, realising that increased confidence, high levels of self-worth/esteem and appropriate support that address barriers to learning make a difference to pupils' learning experiences and their ability to make best use of school provisions. In these schools there is a marked commitment to core principles such as collaboration through pupil voice, senior leadership, ownership, and using the processes and principles of healthy schools to respond to school needs and priorities.

The national programme may not be evident but the concept of healthy schools, places where young people learn about being healthy, where being healthy is modelled within the school, where they become involved and responsible for many aspects of school life, and can see the effect on their learning, lives on.

Healthy schools is sustained because it makes sense to most adults, educationalists, health professionals and parents/carers. Young people themselves see that schools should be the best place to learn about life enhancing skills. Students learn better when they feel safe, happy, healthy and stimulated. This is not difficult to understand. Essentially, healthy schools is about how people lead their lives. In England, the National Healthy Schools Programme was always designed to be fun with considerable emphasis put on celebration and positive relationships.

AUSTRALIA: THE ROLE OF INTERMEDIARY ORGANISATIONS IN THE DEVELOPMENT OF HEALTH PROMOTING SCHOOLS

Louise Rowling and Evie Ledger

Australia is a Commonwealth of eight states and territories. Consequently many challenges arise when implementing new approaches to health and education, as they are both state and national level responsibilities. Policy and funding sources may be from national, state, regional and/or local levels. This complexity of context has shaped the conceptualisation and implementation of health promoting schools. Additionally a unique feature of the context is the existence of the Australian Health Promoting Schools Association (AHPSA). It was created in 1992, on principles drawn from a settings approach (Barry and Dooris, Chapter 2) and an understanding of good health promotion practice being contextual, participatory, multi-strategic and dynamic (Rowling & Jeffreys, 2000). Over the past two decades, AHPSA has provided leadership and made an ongoing contribution to health promoting schools work, that has fostered collaboration, partnerships, knowledge exchange and networking. It is a neutral body representing diverse interests that can advocate in different settings and at all levels of influence (Rowling, 1996). The association's membership base includes teachers, parents, schools and non-government organisations with a common purpose.

A critical feature of the implementation of health promoting schools in Australia compared to some other parts of the world is the existing national level school classroom curriculum, health education, a separate compulsory area of learning. Whereas in other countries, key initial objectives for health promoting schools often focused on developing health curriculum, training teachers and getting health curriculum into the school timetable, in Australia the whole school action often started with policy and environment.

This case study exemplifies how some of the components identified as being necessary for quality school level implementation (Samdal & Rowling, 2011) are equally important to develop and operate in the wider support context at national and state levels. Focus is on policy, partnerships and networking, leadership and sustainability, through description of national activity of AHPSA and two brief state reports exemplifying the components.

Partnerships, networking, leadership and sustainability

AHPSA has played an active role in the development of policy documents. Key documents that were developed were, 'Effective school health promotion: Towards health promoting schools' (National Health and Medical Research Council, 1996) and building on this, the National Strategy for Health Promoting Schools (1997). The former document was written by an expert advisory group, whereas the latter was developed by the Australian Health Promoting Schools Association with funding from the Public Health Division of the Commonwealth Department of Health and Family Services. The strategy was developed drawing on networks across the country, using AHPSA newsletters for raising awareness of the project. AHPSA commissioned four research studies: an audit of school based health promotion; an examination of the nature of health service/school links; an audit of policy and support documents; and a review of priorities for research into health promoting schools in Australia. Information was collected from local, state and national organisations and individuals state and territory consultation, meetings with non-government organisations and agencies and written submissions. The culmination of activity was a National Forum to review results and make recommendations (National Strategy for Health Promoting Schools, 1997). To maximise participation and ownership, raising awareness, network development and capacity building strategies were an integral part of the process of developing the strategy. This seminal document was the first national guideline for policymakers, researchers and practitioners. There were a number of important outcomes of this process. First, the consultative strategy acted as an advocacy process, in that for the first time a national coordinated collaborative report had documented the range of services and support in schools (Stokes & Mukherjee, 2000). Second, as well as building a constituency of supporters, evidence of the varying stages schools and jurisdictions had reached in implementation, was available (Marshall *et al.*, 2000). Third, the results and a description of the collaborative process (Rissel & Rowling, 2000) as well as the results of each of the commissioned research studies were published in a special edition of the *Journal of School Health* (2000: 70(6), 247–261) providing benchmark data and a basis for future growth.

The development of this strategy built partnerships for the association and established networks of people at state, national and global levels. Subsequently, national projects that were influenced by this strategy have been conducted for mental health, physical activity, drug education and sex education (Rowling & Rissel, 2000). A second iteration of the strategy was developed based on the first report, National Framework for Health Promoting Schools (2000–2003). A key focus was developing links between school level activity and national and global policy development. Association activity is ongoing. People continue to come together for conferences; there is collaboration across states and countries, policy level consultation, newsletter, and as technology changed, a dedicated website, list serve and e-documents (http://www.ahpsa.org.au/).

The term 'Intermediary Organisation' has recently emerged principally in implementation science. Cooper (2010) applied this to the educational field, articulating areas of functioning of such organisations namely: linkage and partnerships, policy influence, organisational development, implementation support, capacity building, engagement, accessibility and awareness. The label 'Intermediary Organisation' has not been applied to AHPSA, but the concept encapsulates much of what this organisation has achieved.

A snapshot of the actions emanating from the Health Development Unit, South Australia (now Centre for Health Promotion which is part of SA Health), indicates how functioning as an agency can demonstrate Intermediary Organisation characteristics. The Centre acted as an advocate for health promoting schools and modelled a collaborative style, through its own approach to working 'in and with' school communities. It also linked with ongoing work on Healthy Cities projects and developed joint policy and practice documents with the Education Department. Strong leadership enabled demonstration of agency commitment to health promoting schools and the coordination of partnerships as a priority. There has been organisational and financial support of a grant scheme with its various iterations over many years, as well as the promotion of research and examples of the theory into practice via the 'Virtually Healthy' newsletter, web portal and e-network. In this agency the work with schools and the health promoting schools framework has now merged into health promotion more broadly with no specific school focused activities. This 'absorption' into the core business of an organisation is a positive outcome if the principles and practices have truly been adopted by the organisation.

In New South Wales throughout the early 1990s, individual schools, organ-isations and state Department of Health's health promotion units, had been working on projects, with different entry points such as the setting and specific health topics. Advocacy activity from the state branch of the Health Promoting Schools Association resulted in the production of a document by the state Health Department, 'What Makes a Healthy School Community?' (Renouf, 1992). Building on this, the state Health Department provided leadership and financial support for the production of a comprehensive guide 'Towards a Health Promoting School' (NSW Department of Health & Department of Education, 1996). This was developed jointly with government and non-government educa-tion systems and drafts were widely circulated to different interest groups. Further financial support was provided for implementation of this document, launched jointly by the Ministers for Health and Education. This cross portfolio partnership was rare and proved to be an important agenda setting strategy in the health sector in terms of their relationships with schools. The AHPSA through its conferences also provides opportunities for networking and information exchange between school personnel, health promotion staff and non-government health agencies.

Conclusions

The actions of AHPSA described here, mirroring the brokering function of an 'Intermediary Organisation' have been crucial. Members are mobilised by their common purpose not a particular professional allegiance (Rowling, 1996). In terms of sustainability, health promoting schools is often now referred to as 'a whole school approach' which for the education sector is a more accessible term than health promoting schools. The concept has been absorbed into new projects, for example the MindMatters national mental health promotion framework builds on the three areas of the health promoting schools (http://www.mind matters.edu.au/whole_school_approach/planning_tools/mindmatters_imple mentation_model.html). An opportunity now exists for AHPSA to redevelop its e-network strategy and through this provide ongoing leadership and advocacy for HPS approach. The association is in the process of working towards this, redeveloping their web presence into an online learning community strategy as well as trying to provide an archive of the historical perspective that underpins current progress.

References

Acheson, D. (1998). Independent Inquiry into Inequalities in Health Report. Retrieved from http://www.archive.official-documents.co.uk/document/doh/ih/ih.htm (accessed 21 September 2012).

Black, D. (1980). The Black Report. Retrieved from http://en.wikipedia.org/wiki/ Black_report (accessed 21 September 2012).

Cooper, A. (2010). Knowledge Mobilisation Intermediaries in Education. Retrieved from http://www.oise.utoronto.ca/rspe/UserFiles/File/CSSE2010KMIntermediariesFinal. doc (accessed 21 September 2012).

Marshall, B. J., Sheehan, M. M., Northfield, J. R., Maher, S., Carlisle, R. & Leger, L. H. S. (2000). School-based health promotion across Australia. *Journal of School Health*, *70*(6), 251–252.

National Health and Medical Research Council. (1996). Effective School Health Promotion: Towards Health Promoting Schools. Retrieved from http://www.nhmrc. gov.au/_files_nhmrc/publications/attachments/hp1.pdf (accessed 21 September 2012).

National Strategy for Health Promoting Schools. (1997). National Health Promoting Schools Initiative. Australian Health Promoting Schools Association, from http:// www.ahpsa.org.au/pages/projects.php (accessed 26 January 2012).

NSW Department of Health & Department of Education. (1996). Towards a Health Promoting School. http://catalogue.nla.gov.au/Record/2684444 (accessed 5 April 2012).

Renouf, C. (1992). What Makes a Healthy School Community? NSW Department of Health. http://catalogue.nla.gov.au/Record/2782824 (accessed 5 April 2012).

Rissel, C. & Rowling, L. (2000). Intersectoral collaboration for the development of a national framework for health promoting schools in Australia. *Journal of School Health*, *70*(6), 248–250.

Rowling, L. (1996). The adaptability of the health promoting schools concept: a case study from Australia. *Health Education Research*, *11*(4), 519–526.

Rowling, L. & Jeffreys, V. (2000). Challenges in the development and monitoring of Health Promoting Schools. *Health Education*, *100*, 117–123.

Rowling, L. & Rissel, C. (2000). Impact of the National Health Promoting School Initiative. *Journal of School Health*, *70*(6), 260–261.

Samdal, O. & Rowling, L. (2011). Theoretical and empirical base for implementation components of health promoting schools. *Health Education*, *3*(5), 367–390.

Stokes, H. & Mukherjee, D. (2000). The nature of health service/school links in Australia. *Journal of School Health*, *70*(6), 255–256.

8

PORTUGAL, POLAND AND EUROPE

Preparing and planning for student participation and sustainable health promotion practice at school and national level

In Chapters 4 and 5 preparing and planning for health promotion practice in schools was identified as critical for successful implementation as well as for sustainability. In this chapter two case studies demonstrate how the preparing and planning of the implementation process are important for sustainability both at national level (Portugal) and at local school level (Poland). A systematic process involving the stakeholders in priority of needs and actions is key to the success of the change process. Preparing and planning for the total implementation process also signifies planning for specific components of health promoting schools. A key component of the health promotion approach is the involvement of the target group in terms of student participation. The teachers are the ones to initiate and guide the student participation process. For it to be successful it needs careful planning both at school level and from the individual teacher. The importance of this type of planning is provided through the experiences from a European school-based project on promotion of physical activity and healthy eating.

The Portuguese case study describes a planning process at national level and its importance for sustained action at school level. A working group was established in 2005 by the Ministry of Education, with a mandate to develop a strategy to get all Portuguese schools to include health education as a topic in their curriculum by 2007. After a year the working group made a proposal that health education would be compulsory for schools to include across subjects. This proposal was immediately accepted as public policy and law. The working group continued their strategic planning and next developed a proposal to the government for concrete topic areas to be addressed by schools, which also was accepted as national policy. Following this, the national group identified that guidance was needed to initiate actions at school level. Consequently the working group started to visit schools to help them in their planning and implementation of the health education curriculum. They also continued their planning of more wide reaching support strategies and recommended that the government integrate health promotion in teacher training, both pre-service and in-service. The working group also persuaded the government to provide funding to the schools for implementation of health education and health promoting practice. They proposed the development of a plan for use of the funding be provided before the funding was given. The use of a national working group to develop a strategic plan for implementation of health promotion in schools ensured that health promotion practice did take place at local school level. The economic crisis hit Portugal hard in July 2011 and at the same time PISA results for Maths and Portuguese Language demonstrated that Portuguese students did not perform well in these subjects. Following a change of minister, the health promotion focus was taken off the priority list, and no support or encouragement are now given to the schools, thereby dramatically threatening the sustainability of health promotion in Portuguese schools.

The Polish case study presents concrete steps of how to plan for successful implementation of health promotion practice at school level. The planning process described includes three stages: (1) preparation, (2) diagnosis of needs, and (3) planning of action and its evaluation. These stages are preceded by the implementation and evaluation stages. These five stages normally represent a working cycle of one to three years. Each stage has three or more steps, all of which have been developed in close collaboration with schools and are currently used by all schools that enter established regional networks of health promoting schools. An important motivation for the development of the concrete planning guidelines was the observation that schools in the early phase of the national health promoting school network spent too little time on planning and initiated lots of actions that did not always have clear aims and objectives for what change to obtain. The preparation stage aims to raise commitment for the health promoting school practice, and build motivation to participate among staff and partners of collaboration. The stage of diagnosis includes a systematic collection of data and perceived needs for change from students, teachers, parents and collaborators. The data collection could be done through interviews or surveys. By using this approach the school has a basis for taking decisions on which aims to set for their health promotion practice, i.e. what they need to change and improve. This is addressed in the third planning stage, planning of action. In this stage, concrete steps for how to identify priorities of aims as well as actions that can solve or improve the prioritised area are developed. A key issue of the prioritisation is that the school should focus and limit their actions so that they have the capacity to maintain the agreed actions over time and also to better target their aim for change.

To demonstrate the importance of preparing and planning for student participation a two-year project in 19 European countries focusing on healthy eating and physical activity, using student involvement through action oriented change as the key strategy, is presented. Student participation was based on issues in students' everyday lives and on dialogue and negotiation, with each other and with teachers. For this process to be effective teachers were given guidance to act as facilitators, inspiring, supporting and challenging students. The project identified three different functions that participation achieved: motivating, influencing and as a teaching and learning strategy. Students' authentic responsibility opportunities resulted in developing a sense of ownership, which is the key aim of involving the target group in health promotion. However, results of the project found that to effectively build the capacities of teachers and students, specific guidance and support was needed, demonstrating the need to prepare and plan for successful student participation.

ADOLESCENTS' HEALTH EDUCATION AND PROMOTION IN PORTUGAL: A CASE STUDY OF PLANNING FOR SUSTAINABLE PRACTICE

Margarida Gaspar de Matos, Daniel Sampaio, Isabel Baptista and Equipa Aventura Social, UTL and CMDT/UNL

Introduction

This case study aims to describe how a ministerial process that took place in Portugal in 2005 (The GTES Ministerial Group) was able to revitalise health promotion in Portugal and achieve positive and sustainable results. The text will explore sustainability through addressing the core questions of 'to what extent is health promotion sufficiently and adequately integrated and anchored in the Portuguese educational system, and/or do circumstantial factors such as economic restrictions or changing educational priorities prevent sustainability?'

The educational system in Portugal

In the 1960s the first 'School Health' programme was introduced in Portugal, although limited to (a few) medical interventions and restricted to children who attended school. In the early 1990s the programme 'Viva la Escola' ('Let the school live') (1990–1993) was established, followed immediately by the Portuguese Network of Health Promoting Schools (RNEPS) integrated in the European network (ENHPS) (1995–2003). The aim of the European network was to move health promotion in school beyond 'project status' and get it fully embedded in the regular dynamic of each European school. In Portugal joining the network was a milestone coinciding with a tough period of political turbulence, with four government changes in a four year period. It was only in 2005 that this process was remodelled, revitalised and pushed forward.

Preparing and planning for school development

In mid-2005, the Ministry of Education decided to change health education in Portuguese schools into a regular, long lasting, sustainable process. A Working Group for Health Education (GTES – Grupo de Trabalho para a Educação Sexual/ Educação para a Saúde) was established. The aim was to develop proposals, for schools all over the country, to include health education in their curriculum, by the year 2007.

The GTES team started its activities in June 2005 and by the end of the year it proposed that health education should be compulsory in schools, across all school subjects, calling for students' and parents' active participation. This proposal was immediately accepted as public policy and law. Later on, four main health issues for priority intervention were identified: (1) Substance use; (2) Sexuality/IST and HIV prevention; (3) Nutrition and physical activity, and (4) Violence prevention and well-being/mental health. GTES published three reports, in 2005 and 2007 that were the basis for all national legislation in the area from 2007 until 2011 (http://www. dgidc.min-edu.pt/educacaosaude/index.php?s=directorio&pid=107, retrieved 10.08.2011).

During the GTES mandated period the GTES group visited local projects in numerous schools all over Portugal and organised various national and regional meetings for teachers, principals and experts in health promotion, in order to establish a participatory platform for sustained action. GTES also provided planning, supervision, and evaluation action in schools, through their visits and meetings across the country. Several participants from the local community were invited to the meetings. Networking and re-organisation of school and local health services and resources were identified as a priority. In particular, biology and physical education teachers, as well as psychologists, nurses, social workers and school medical doctors were encouraged and expected to collaborate.

Policy and institutional anchoring

Following GTES recommendations, the law No. 25 995/2005, 16 December, defined health education as compulsory in schools and nominated a teacher in every national school as the 'Health Coordinator'. In each school there is a school educational plan that includes Health Education for all and defines schools as healthy and friendly environments (Law 2506/2007, 20 February). After the first GTES report in 2005, a protocol between the Ministry of Education and the Ministry of Health was signed, in order to stimulate better interaction between schools and local health centres, and a responsible person (a medical doctor) was appointed by the Ministry of Health from each health centre. Close collaboration was also carried on with local authorities in the local communities.

Professional development and learning

The issue of teacher training was raised and addressed in a threefold way. First, the Ministry of Education should organise specific training for 'health promotion' especially regarding the four main health issues, beginning with specific training for the school nominated 'coordinator of health promotion interventions'.

Second, the universities and pedagogical institutes were encouraged to integrate health promotion training in the pre-service teacher training programmes. Third, they were encouraged to offer specialisation by means of master and doctoral study programmes in 'health promotion'. All the training approaches were meant to include 'specific health information/knowledge' but with the overall training in active listening and group dynamics, to increase pupils' participation in active and interactive health sessions.

Sustainability

GTES recommended that, after a round of applications demonstrating a plan for use of the funding and use of cost–benefit evaluations, a permanent grant be awarded to every school on an annual basis. Some schools argued for a recurrent special budget allocation avoiding bureaucracy and delays in the attribution of funds to projects making planning and sustainability hard to manage. Furthermore, it was argued the grant should be independent of government changes. For example, during the school year 2010–2011 the budget allocated to the schools was suddenly made dependent on priority given to training teachers in sexual education. This measure was defined at a central level in agreement with the regional level.

More than 2,200 teachers were under training in Sexual education: active and participative methodologies in sexual education, whereas other areas have not been given this priority.

In a final part of this implementation process back in the middle of 2010, further legislation papers were promulgated and published, outlining continued countrywide implementation of health promotion, the adequacy of the process was already established, the training of professionals was carried out, and a few indicators of positive change were achieved; major financial, human and physical resources being already allocated.

However, in July 2011 the economic crisis had a severe impact on the situation. At the same time the PISA results for Maths and Portuguese Language were considered so low that the new Minister of Education decided that these two subjects should be the new priority focus for academic reinforcement and thereby replacing the previous 'non-disciplinary curricular areas' up till then devoted to health promotion. For the moment the 'health promotion process' is therefore interrupted or at least no longer a national priority thus seriously compromising the sustainability. However, some optimism is possible in regard to the new curricular organisation for the school year 2011–2012 (Decree – Law no. 50//2011, 9 April and Decree – Law no. 94/2011, 3 August) where 'Citizenship education' is the only 'non disciplinary curricular area'. It is compulsory and the schools are obliged to cover 'the education for health and education for citizenship'. One school year has 33–36 sessions of citizenship education: 12 sessions of the total must be integrated into education for health – sexual education.

Reflections on what has contributed to and threatened sustainability

The substantial planning and national anchoring process following the establishment of the GTES working group seems to have been an essential basis for the rapid growth of health promotion efforts in Portuguese schools. Integrating the expected actions as part of national laws obliged schools to address health promotion and health education, although it was left to the schools to identify how to meet the national expectations, i.e. in which subject/topic areas to include the new activities. No allocation of curriculum time seems to have been a threat to the priority given by the schools, and the actual implementation thereby became dependent on the principal's allocation of resources and priority to health education and promotion. Furthermore, the unclear role of health education in the national evaluation process performed for each school was an additional ambiguity.

The regional and national initiatives towards teacher training also positively influenced what happened at the individual school as these processes took place independently of the principal's priority. The importance of national and regional initiatives is further demonstrated by the abrupt change in national priorities in July 2011. This change in expectations and priorities from the national government is likely to negatively influence the priority given to health education and health promotion at individual schools, particularly seen in contrast to the previous strong national support for the topic area.

PREPARING AND PLANNING FOR THE HEALTH PROMOTING SCHOOLS DEVELOPMENT IN POLAND

Barbara Woynarowska

Introduction

In 1992, Poland became a member of the European Network of Health Promoting Schools and the first regional network was also established in that year. Regional networks now exist in all regions. This case study reports on findings from schools involved, with a particular focus on the preparing and planning component of implementation. The guidelines for implementation of HPS were developed with participation of school coordinators in Poland during the pilot project (1992–1995). These guidelines, published as manuals (Woynarowska & Sokołowska, 2000) are currently used, with some modification, in all regional networks. According to these guidelines schools are encouraged to follow a cycle of five stages:

1. Preparation:

    • initiation;
    • first information for school community;
    • explanation of the HPS concept;
    • looking for partners and supporters;
    • creation of the structure supporting health promotion activities.

2. Diagnosis of initial situation:

    • collection of data concerning current problems of school community;
    • analysis of these data;
    • list of priorities (problems/needs).

3. Planning of action (intervention) and its evaluation:

    • establish priority/priorities (for action);
    • analysis of reasons for selected priority problem and defining the method of their reduction/elimination;
    • defining aim/s of action;
    • build the plan for action and plan for evaluation.

4. Implementation of the plan and process of evaluation.
5. Outcomes evaluation.

This cycle is repeated every school year, although the preparatory stage only involves new members of a school community. This annual process is found to be more useful than developing a plan for a longer time period as the rhythm of school activity is defined by the school year. The present case study describes the first three stages.

Stage 1. Preparation

The aim of Stage One is to prepare members of the school community to make the decision and start to implement the HPS concept in their school. The duration of this stage is about six to eight months, depending on the specific school's situation. This stage includes the following five steps.

Step 1. Initiation

Aim: to create the initiation group and identify a leader and a few people who are interested in the HPS concept. The initiation group should:

- gain basic knowledge of the HPS and understand its concept and criteria;
- ask themselves: What are the needs and expectations of our school? What will be the benefits and disadvantage of changes introduced? Can we do this?
- identify other people (including member of the school management) interested in this concept and ready to disseminate and support its implementation.

Step 2. First information to school community

Aim: to disseminate information about planned initiative, through discussion in different groups, providing a basis for prioritising activities. The prioritising of activities will be informed by a survey conducted among staff, students and parents. The following simple questionnaire is distributed to teachers, non-teaching staff, pupils and parents to complete anonymously.

WHAT INFLUENCES MY WELL-BEING AT SCHOOL?

1. Very positively:
2. Positively:
3. Rather positively:
4. Negatively:

Step 3. Explanation of the HPS concept

Aim: to help the whole school community to understand the HPS concept. Participation of all stakeholders (staff, students and parents) is a core element. Health promotion is most likely a new idea for the school community, and the creation of the HPS is a long process that requires implementation of new approaches and methods. It is recommended that the leader or initiation group organises workshops for different groups of stakeholders (teachers, students, parents). Together they should look for answers to the following questions:

- What does 'being healthy' mean and what affects health?
- What does the health promoting school mean?
- What are the most important criteria of the HPS?
- Where is our school according these criteria?

Step 4. Looking for partners and supporters

Aim: to disseminate the HPS concept and plan for development among parents and some partners in the local community. This may be done by the leader or initiation group. It is important to address: Why is the creation of the HPS important for our school? What would be the benefits? It is recommended that an event be organised for parents and the local community. The aim of the event is to invite parents and the local community to discuss planned actions in a relaxed atmosphere.

Step 5. Creation of the structure supporting health promotion activities

Aim: to appoint a school coordinator and team for the health promotion initiative:

- The roles of the school coordinator should be a volunteer, elected demo-cratically and should have:
  - a position in school enabling influence on school policy and decision making (ideally it is the headteacher or his/her deputy);
  - personal characteristics enabling efficient and healthy functioning (preventing burn-out due to increased workload) and should also have good interpersonal skills;
  - readiness for professional as well as personal and social development and change, for example by making health promoting changes in his/her own lifestyle.
- The tasks of the school coordinator as well as rules and regulations of cooperation between the school coordinator with the headmaster and the rest of the school HPS team should be defined.
- *The health promoting school team* consists of representatives from different groups of the school community: teachers, non-teaching staff, students, parents, school nurse and people from the local community. Belonging to the team is voluntary. Members of the team should have good knowledge and understanding of the HPS concept, and be enthusiastic, active, creative and supportive towards the school coordinator. The rules of the team's activities should be clearly defined. An important task is to document the activities of the school coordinator and school team.

Stage 2. Diagnosis of initial situation

Aims:

- to identify the real problems (needs) of the school community;
- to summarise what was done until now ('no school is at a 0 point');
- to collect objective data which will be used in the stage of final self-evaluation of the undertaken projects.

Expected outcome: a list of problems which should be solved. This creates a basis for selection of priority problem/s for intervention. *The selection is made jointly* by the school coordinator and school health promotion team.

How to perform the diagnosis? On the basis of experiences within the project two types of diagnosis are proposed:

- *General, complex diagnosis*: Large scale survey using established measures. This diagnosis approach is complicated and time consuming.
- *Partial, stage related diagnosis*: Each school year the simplistic questionnaire presented earlier is given to the stakeholders. The survey should be complemented by discussions, observations, and documents.

Stage 3 Planning of action (intervention) and its evaluation

Experiences from the pilot project showed that planning was a 'weak side' of many schools. The guidelines for school coordinators were therefore developed based on publications and consultancy of Leo Barić (1994), figure 8.1.

The basic principles of planning

- Planning should be *realistic.*
- *Small steps* – no more than one or two aims, recognised as priorities.
- *Many people* should participate in choice of priorities.
- The plan should be a result of consultation with the school community, parents, and representatives of the local community and the final plan should be presented to them.
- Planning of activities *is connected to* planning of process and outcome evaluation.
- Plan relates to a determined period of time – e.g. one school year.

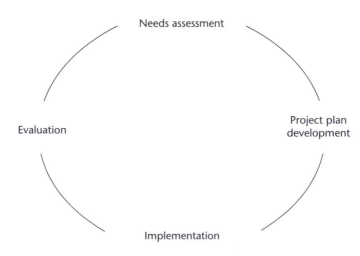

FIGURE 8.1 Planning model based on Barić (1994)

Planning is a *process* consisting of an initial stage and then building a plan of activities

1. Initial stage of planning

The planning process starts with an initial stage, which precedes diagnosis of initial state (baseline data collection). The aim of this stage is to choose the *priority problem*, to recognise its *causes* and to find the *solutions for removing* these causes.

Step 1. Establishment of the list of problems. Based on the diagnosis in the initial stage of a list of problems.

Step 2. Choice of priorities. The list of problems in a school is usually very long. Priorities are needed.

- *Criteria for choosing priorities.* According to the school specific situation the following can be considered:

  - frequent occurrence;
  - the rank of the problem;
  - its specific arduousness or danger;
  - ease of achieving aims;
  - availability of resources.

- *How to choose priorities.* As many people as possible should participate in the prioritisation process. Being actively involved in the whole process assists commitment.

Step 3. Recognition of the causes of selected priority. This is a task for the school coordinator and school team on health promotion or other group (depending on school). The following method of activity is suggested:

- identification of all possible causes of selected priority;
- selection of cause which might be: the most important, most probable, realistic to remove;
- determination of the *main cause(s)* out of selected causes.

Step 4. Finding solutions for removing the causes of the problem. This stage uses the same method of activity as step 3:

- identification;
- solutions;
- determination of the *final solution(s)*, the starting point to establish tasks of planned work.

2. Building the plan of activities and their evaluation

The plan has to be built and written precisely and clearly, so it enables *process*

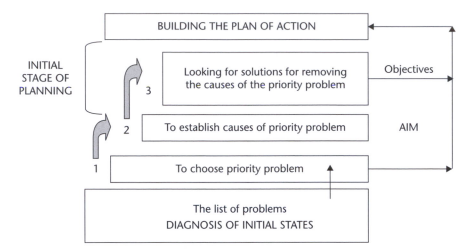

FIGURE 8.2   Scheme of a stage of planning and its link with diagnosis of initial state and building the plan of action

and outcomes evaluation. The most useful way to write the plan is presented in the table below. The plan should be clear in its form and it should be presented to school and local communities. It should contain the following elements:

Elements of the plan

1 Aim

1. Define criteria for success.
2. The method of assessment of the achievements (success):
   a. What shows that the aim has been achieved (indicators)?
   b. How to assess if the aim has been achieved (tools)?
   c. Who assesses when that the aim has been achieved?

2 Objectives

1. Define criteria for success.
2. Identify methods of implementation.
3. Describe people involved.
4. List resources.
5. The method of assessment of implementation of activities:
   a. What shows that activities have been implemented (indicators)?
   b. How to assess if activities have been implemented (tools)?
   c. Who assesses when the activities have been implemented?

Conclusions

Implementation of the cycle of five stages described earlier, developed over one to three years is the basis for schools to apply to become a member of the regional network of health promoting schools. A survey on understanding and acceptance of the HPS concepts by the school community and the implementation of planning and evaluation procedures are also carried out by schools that want to apply for the Health Promoting School National Certificate.

STUDENT PARTICIPATION AS AN IMPORTANT DIMENSION OF THE HEALTH PROMOTING SCHOOL: EXPERIENCE FROM A EUROPEAN PROJECT

Venka Simovska

Introduction

This case study considers the participatory approach employed in the European project '*Shape Up: A school-community approach to influence the determinants of a healthy and balanced growing up*'[1]. Shape Up ran during the period 2006–2008 in 19 cities in 19 EU countries. In total, 73 schools, 2,300 students, and 140 teachers were involved, assisted by 38 local coordinators and facilitators and five international competence centres.

Key components in the implementation

The fundamental premise of the Shape Up approach was that healthy lifestyles are influenced in sustainable ways by addressing their determinants at the school, family, community, and broader societal levels, rather than solely at an individual behaviour level. Based on this premise, the project aimed to bring together the principles of participatory health education, prevention, and health promotion in an integrated intervention programme, in this case focused on the specific health topics of healthy eating and physical activity.

The methodological framework was embedded within the health promoting schools principles. The following assumptions provided the basis for the methodological framework (Simovska, 2007):

- Student participation and ownership are key elements of the approach.
- Participation needs to be carefully planned and guided.
- Action-oriented knowledge about health can be gained through participation in authentic, real life health promoting actions in school (Simovska, 2007).
- Action-oriented knowledge is multidisciplinary and multidimensional (Jensen, 1997).

- The Investigation–Vision–Action–Change (IVAC) approach (Jensen, 1997) is a beneficial model to structure action–oriented participation in school context.
- Collaboration between school and local community fosters a range of opportunities.

Consistent with the main underlying principles, the project methodological approach was characterised by the following features.

Student involvement

The participating students were actively involved in deciding about specific issues within the area of healthy eating and physical activity that they wished to investigate. Moreover, they were engaged in deciding about strategies to be used to explore these issues as well as in representing and communicating their findings and reflections. These decision making processes were based on a dialogue and negotiation among the students and between the students and teachers, aimed at constructing and clarifying meanings and values relating to the health issues in question. An essential part of the dialogue and decision making process in this regard was a discussion of the significance of the issues to students' everyday lives.

Action and change focus

The project was directed towards taking action and initiating health promoting change with regard to the overall project topics. The action-focused teaching emphasises the importance of close collaboration between the school and the local community. Each action needed a clear goal, that is, it should represent an attempt by the students to bring about positive change relating to the health problem in question. The change could be in students' and adults' attitudes, knowledge and critical awareness about the problem but also in health-related conditions in the school or the local environment, i.e. in the social determinants of the problem on a proximal level. Students' ideas, previous knowledge and their lived experience should play crucial roles with regard to which changes and actions were to be carried out.

Pedagogical design

The IVAC (Investigation-Vision-Action-Change) (Jensen, 1997) approach was employed as the main common framework for structuring and facilitating student participation. The approach was modified and adjusted to fit the specifics of each particular context and the existing systems of meaning characterising the school culture in each of the participating countries. Furthermore, the approach was adapted to the personal understanding, professional skills, preferences and experience of the participating teachers, project facilitators and coordinators. Within this approach teachers and other project staff had the role of responsible facilitators of the project activities with the tasks of inspiring, supporting and challenging the students. They engaged in the educational dialogue with the students, with an aim of broadening the health concepts and health related knowledge to include the social dimensions, international perspectives, equity and democratic values as well as specific strategies for management of health promoting change on school and local community levels.

Context and different ways of implementing participation

The implementation of Shape Up took different forms in each of the participating schools, depending on the specifics of the broader (i.e. cultural, educational and societal) and immediate context (e.g. each school's priorities for health promotion, conditions, and resources). Acknowledging the complexity and the dynamic nature of each particular context, the project aimed to utilise this by applying the Internet and cross-cultural collaboration and by providing a shared 'virtual' context. This was conceived of as the interplay of the local systems of meaning with the overall theoretical foundation and the common project framework developed through a dialogue between the researchers and the participating teachers, facilitators and local stakeholders.

Three main forms of participation were identified across the different local contexts:

1. Participation as a *motivation* strategy, characterised by involving students in project activities whose content and structure were determined by the adults, sometimes in consultation with students. Students were involved in choosing one among a few pre-determined activities; for example, some schools offered several new forms of physical activity and students could select which ones they preferred to be included in regular PE classes.
2. Participation as a *teaching-learning* strategy characterised by a scaffold-like pedagogical approach which involved providing close guidance to ensure students' learning through experiences of success, for example in selecting and prioritising the health promoting actions at the school or in the local environment surrounding the school.
3. Participation as an *influence* strategy characterised by students having a genuine influence over the decisions about the health promoting actions to be undertaken in the project. Within the given frames of the project topic, healthy eating and physical activity, students were guided by the project staff to decide on specific health promoting changes they would like to bring about, and to take action to realise these changes. Examples include establishing a new playground near the school, or changing the menu at the school cafeteria, planned and brought about by students themselves.

Conclusions and challenges

In conclusion, it could be argued that even though the overall project topics were decided outside of the project's frames and were assigned to students, the students investigated the area in their own ways, guided by their teachers and using the broad possibilities of the Internet and cross-cultural collaboration. The focus of the participation was on processes of critical reflection, goal-oriented dialogue and negotiation of meanings related to health matters rather than students acquiring a factual body of knowledge and moulding students' lifestyles. However, the fact that the students shared the responsibility for selecting aspects of the topics to be investigated and methods they would use to do so resulted in an increased sense of ownership. This led further to increased student intent and responsibility, which contributed to building better understanding and competence to take action to promote health.

Research in relation to the project pointed out that adequate student guidance from teachers and other adults is central to the effectiveness of this approach. However, participatory and change-oriented work seem to pose a number of challenges for schools, especially when the curriculum is not flexible enough to allow for modifications of content and pedagogy, and when the wider context is largely unresponsive to children as agents of change. These challenges are:

- Transferring the project-based principles into regular health promoting school curriculum, which would take account of students' concepts, concerns and everyday experience in relation to health in their social contexts, including the social, structural, cultural and other aspects related to health.
- Establishing effective collaboration structures between schools and local governance in order to ensure space for students' participation and influence.
- Lack of support for teachers, particularly in terms of new ways of providing balance between open classroom discourse and guiding students through the broad health-knowledge and health promotion landscape.
- Providing an appropriate balance between institutional needs – for instance for control, health improvement and safety – and the genuine views of students on their needs in relation to health. In other words, addressing the issue of choice in relation to health that the school authorities may not wish to have on the premises and yet the students may have expectations that such a choice is available to them in participatory work, e.g. vending machines selling sweet carbonated drinks or confectionery.
- Facilitating school change so that the participatory and action-oriented health promoting school is conducive to informing policy agendas with young people's ideas, needs and visions concerning health and well-being.

Note

1 The project was co-financed by the EC, DG SANCO. More about the project's organisational structure and funding is available on shapeupeurope.net.

References

Barić, L. (1994). *Health Promotion and Health Education in Practice. Module 2: The Organisational Model*. Altrincham: Barns Publications.

Jensen, B. B. (1997). A case of two paradigms within health education. *Health Education Research*, *12*(4), 419–428.

Simovska, V. (2007). The changing meanings of participation in school based health education and health promotion. *Health Education Research*, *22*(6), 864–878.

Woynarowska B., Sokołowska M. (2000) Poland: the Health-Promoting School National certificate, In: C. V. Whitman, C. E. Aldinger (eds), *Case Studies in Global School Health Promotion. From Research to Practice*. New York: Springer, pp. 214–224.

9

GERMANY AND SCOTLAND

Partnership and networking

In Chapters 4 and 5, partnership and networking was identified as a key component for successful implementation of health promoting schools. This chapter presents two case studies addressing the importance of partnership and networking at national level and at regional and local level. The partnership and networking between the health and education sector and between stake-holders' organisations (ministries, schools, NGOs) and individuals (ministers, principals, teachers, parents and students) opened doors to discuss and define how health promoting schools can also contribute to achieve educational goals. This common understanding was core to the priority and thereby the success of the implementation.

The German case study describes the influence of a national alliance in getting both national school authorities and local schools to give priority to health promotion. The alliance includes ministries and organisations relating to health and education matters and individual students, teachers and parents who have an interest in health promoting schools. The driving force of the alliance is to advocate that health promoting schools also promote educational learning through the concept of a 'good healthy school'. The alliance represents an important arena for decisions makers to meet to discuss and listen to arguments and develop their understanding for the importance of health promotion for educational learning. The alliance has developed support material for schools to use when they want to implement health promoting schools. It also aims to support federal states in their efforts to improve education quality in schools. In 2008 the alliance became a formal organisation and continues its systematic support structure for national, regional and local levels.

The Scottish case study describes the development of a partnership between the education and health sectors and how, when this was formalised in 2002, it represented the breakthrough of placing health promoting schools on the local school agenda. Much effort was put into the establishment and maintenance of the partnership to ensure that it was built on trust and shared values and commitments. The systematic focus on partnerships and also on giving autonomy to local authorities in the implementation of health promoting schools is described as a key success factor for the full integration of health promoting schools in the new curriculum, 'Curriculum for Excellence', in 2004. In this curriculum health promotion is part of the school's obligation as for any other subject area and is also included in the national audits of each school.

GERMANY: ANSCHUB.DE – ALLIANCE FOR SUSTAINABLE SCHOOL HEALTH AND EDUCATION

Kevin Dadaczynski and Peter Paulus

Current situation and driving forces in school health promotion in Germany

The administrative responsibility for educational and health issues in German schools falls within the jurisdiction of each of the 16 federal states (Ministries of Education). Thus, no uniform regulations are in place on education and health. However, on the basis of its regulations, and anchored in school laws, each federal state oversees the statutory task of 'health education', which is quite different between each federal state. The evaluation of the dissemination of the health promoting school approach in Germany revealed that only 14 per cent of German schools had adopted a whole school approach to health (Paulus & Witteriede, 2008). As a result of this and due to other developments (e.g. the results of the Programme for International Student Assessment, PISA) the so-called 'good healthy school' approach as an innovative concept to school health promotion has been developed in recent years (Paulus, 2005). This approach takes into account that, first, schools are mainly legitimised by their educational and not by health responsibilities and that, second, health can contribute to strengthening academic outcomes (e.g. Suhrcke & de Paz Nieves, 2011) and the overall quality of education. Within this approach health is seen as a key driver for school quality. Hence, a 'good healthy school' supports the realisation of its educational mission by applying health related measures. A key driver of the development, implementation, and dissemination of this approach and its accompanying programme Anschub.de was the strong financial support from the German Bertelsmann-Foundation.

Anschub.de

Anschub.de, an alliance for sustainable school health and education in Germany, was the first project of the 'good healthy school' approach on a national level, which was developed and piloted from 2002 to 2010 by the Bertelsmann-Foundation. The programme is aimed at all people involved in the school including pupils, teachers, parents but also, and in particular, the bodies responsible for the school such as school administrations and education and health ministries. The overall goal of Anschub.de is to sustainably empower schools to systematically improve their educational quality through structured and evidence based health actions (Paulus, 2009). To achieve this goal, Anschub.de has produced a set of 13 modules to support the implementation of the programme. It is currently applied by four out of 16 federal states with a total of nine networks encompassing more than 200 schools, 70,000 pupils and 5,500 teachers. Evaluation results indicate that schools that participated in the programme report significant improvements in all dimensions of school quality over a three-year period, with highest effect sizes for pupils (Paulus & Gediga, 2010).

The following case study will focus on two implementation factors (Partnership and networking; Sustainability) that we perceive to be well addressed within Anschub.de.

Partnership and networking

From the beginning, within Anschub.de, a national level alliance of about 40 stakeholders was developed. This alliance encompasses organisations from various societal fields who believe they have a responsibility for educational and health matters (e.g. ministries of education, health and accident assurance companies, teacher training institutes, drug-abuse prevention agencies, national associations of pupils and parents, and a professional organisation of architects). In Germany this way of partnering reflects a new way of thinking and allowed decision makers from various societal fields to discuss and work together to promote the health, well-being and educational quality. The alliance included the development of a position paper about the basic understanding of an integrated approach to school health promotion and education within Anschub.de, as well as support activities in school health promotion at the regional or local level. In addition to the national alliance, so-called 'educational landscapes', that are regional in scope, were established. Each 'educational landscape' consisted of a network of schools (the more heterogeneous the better), which were supported by regional governmental and non-governmental organisations. All participating schools cooperated to translate the vision of a 'good healthy school' into practice. They were coordinated by a local or regional steering group with representatives from the school and local and/or regional organisations.

Additionally, supervision and support were provided by a coordinator appointed for each region. Using existing structures, the regional coordinators typically came from school related positions such as school development, school psychology or directly from the school. They were appointed by Ministries of Education and trained in school health development and networking of clusters of good healthy schools. The cooperation is guided by target agreements (e.g.

raising the psychosocial school climate) and project structure plans (e.g. defining aims, objectives and measurements) which were signed with each federal state or region. Finally, the involvement of parents is of the utmost importance within Anschub.de. To facilitate this, parents were involved in periodical evaluations of the school and its educational quality. Furthermore, specific materials were developed and evaluated which helped schools to promote parental involvement. One instrument used in this context is the so-called 'climate conference' which aims to facilitate parents to exchange views about a certain school topic. Step by step, the parents chose specific projects and initiatives during the course of the climate conference to bring them into the school community.

Sustainability

The 'good healthy school' approach can be understood as a step towards sustainability as it links health and education in an innovative way. If schools begin to understand that health can promote educational quality, it can be expected that they do not see health as an additional task but as a regular part of the school mission. If that is attained, it becomes possible that school health is more than a project limited to a couple of weeks. Schools which take part in Anschub.de run through a typical planning and implementation cycle which encompasses different stages. In Anschub.de the problem analysis is focused on the assessment of both school and educational quality by using a self evaluation instrument, SEIS – self evaluation in schools (Stern, Ebel, Vaccaro & Vorndran, 2006).

Although this self evaluation procedure is comprehensive and requires the commitment of all people involved in the school (pupils, teachers, and parents), it reduces extra efforts that would possibly arise when exclusively focusing on health. The regional 'educational landscapes' are composed in a way that supports sustainability through exchange of experiences and creating partnerships with other schools and, importantly, with local organisations that can support them permanently in becoming a 'good healthy school'. Professional development is acknowledged to be an important aspect of capacity building and hence of sustainability (NSW Health Department, 2001). Anschub.de has developed specific modules for the training of coordinators, qualifying them for networking and supporting schools, teams of teachers, parents, pupils, and others involved in the development of a good healthy school.

Finally, it is worth noting that Anschub.de became a formal association in 2008 acting as a national platform for health and education. The main aim of the association (www.anschub.de) is to disseminate the 'good healthy school' approach and to support current initiatives and projects within the federal states. All materials developed in the pilot phase are freely accessible on the association's website. Furthermore, Anschub.de as an association aims to influence the political level with the Berlin declaration on health and education adopted at the end of 2010. This declaration appeals to all relevant societal players to further develop and disseminate the concept of 'good healthy schools'.

Reflection on barriers and challenges

One challenge within Anschub.de was to overcome conflicting intentions of the alliance partners and to establish a structure that enabled synergistic effects. To address this, three forum meetings were organised right at the beginning, which aimed to create a shared understanding of relevant problems in the field of school health promotion. Furthermore, an economic evaluation of partnering with Anschub.de was performed. Results indicate that it paid off (in economic terms) for each partner to be part of the alliance. Another challenge was to establish a regional steering group for each 'educational landscape' and to motivate them to keep on working. To identify partners who have an impact in that region, who are interested in cooperation with each other and build an alliance at the regional level was one of the important tasks to be solved by the coordinators. Since 2008 sustainability of Anschub.de has been challenged by the need to seek funding from other sources.

FROM HEALTH TO EDUCATION: THE JOURNEY TOWARDS HEALTH PROMOTING SCHOOL IMPLEMENTATION IN SCOTLAND

Jo Inchley, Lisa Gugglberger and Ian Young

Introduction

This case study focuses on the process of implementation of health promoting schools (HPS) in Scotland. The health promotion sector in Scotland was among the early developers and early adopters of the concept internationally in the 1980s (Young and Williams, 1989) and the case study identifies the key events, actors, policies and processes which have facilitated its progress to date. It focuses specifically on the need for political anchoring and effective partnership working in order to support sustainable outcomes. From the early days of innovation within the health sector, the health promoting school concept has now been formally embedded within the education system through a new curriculum, 'Curriculum for Excellence', which was introduced in 2010.

The political context

Scotland is part of the United Kingdom, with a population of 5.2 million. The Scottish Parliament was established in 1999 giving Scotland more control over its own affairs. Although Scotland has always had a separate education system and traditions, health and education were formally confirmed as devolved powers. Since devolution, there has been a shift from highly centralised forms of policy-making to a more decentralised form, paying more attention to processes of consultation (Grek, 2011).

Policy and institutional anchoring at national and local school level

At the end of the 1990s two important documents were published which highlighted the importance of the HPS in moving beyond a traditional health education model to a more holistic understanding of the role of schools in promoting health: (1) the Health White Paper, 'Towards a Healthier Scotland' (Scottish Office, 1999); and (2) curricular guidelines for schools 'Health Education 5–14' (Learning and Teaching Scotland, 1999). These documents, one from the health sector and one from the education sector, provided a platform for national HPS implementation. Subsequently, a ministerial commitment was made to take action and establish a unit to oversee HPS development across Scotland and a national target was set for all schools to become health promoting schools by 2007 (Scottish Executive, 2003).

The Scottish Health Promoting Schools Unit (SHPSU) was established in 2002 and, importantly, was located within the education sector with support from both the health and education ministries and the national health promotion agency. This was a crucial step forward in mainstreaming and establishing HPS in the education sector (Young & Currie, 2009). It provided national leadership, coordination and support for all partners to develop health promoting schools throughout Scotland. Recent research supports the view that the unit was crucial in establishing HPS implementation and in sustaining the partnership between health, education and central government, although establishing these partnerships was not always an easy process (Gugglberger, 2011). Developing effective partnerships requires building of trust, developing mutual under-standing (language, concepts, values), agreeing on budget commitments and responsibilities, and accepting challenges to traditional professional roles (Young & Lee, 2009).

A national framework, 'Being well – doing well' (SHPSU, 2004), was published which provided a vision for health promoting schools in Scotland and set out key values, aims and characteristics. Local authorities, in partnership with local NHS Health Boards, were given responsibility for developing their own accreditation framework against which to measure progress towards the national target. The results of this process were heterogeneous with considerable diversity in the approaches taken. However, all local authorities were required to create a body of evidence and state how they would ensure that all schools were health promoting schools, so that their accreditation frameworks were endorsed nation-ally. Giving power to local authorities in this way was part of a general strategy to allow greater autonomy at regional level and thus to further local solutions to local issues. The need for flexibility and bottom-up solutions was seen as critical to success.

A similar need for flexibility and responsiveness to local needs was evident in an earlier school case study research (Inchley & Currie, 2003). Here, a broad focus on healthy eating was pre-determined but schools were given the autonomy and scope to decide how to take this forward according to their own needs and local context. It was clear that school staff were more likely to engage with the project when it was 'rooted in the school'. Such a sense of ownership can, in turn, promote a 'can-do' attitude to change (Koelen, Vaandrager & Colomer, 2001) and is crucial to successful implementation.

Institutional anchoring was also highly dependent on school management and the existence of key staff or 'champions' to drive the work forward. The involvement of the Head Teacher or other member of school management was critical to effective implementation through giving status to the project and allocating the necessary time and resources (Inchley, Muldoon & Currie, 2007).

Mainstreaming within education – a sustainable approach to health and well-being

In 2007, the Schools (Health Promotion and Nutrition) Scotland Act was passed by the Scottish Parliament, giving local authorities statutory responsibility for ensuring that Scottish schools were health promoting and, for the first time, that food and drink served in schools met nutritional standards. NHS Health Boards were recognised as key partners in the development and implementation of the Act. With HPS more fully established in education policy and practice, the national unit was disbanded in 2008 and its role subsumed by the national agency for education and learning. This heralded a new phase of HPS implementation in which health promoting schools became fully embedded in the education system, with the implementation of a new curriculum, 'Curriculum for Excellence' (Scottish Executive, 2004), and the mainstreaming of 'health and well-being' in Scottish schools. This latest development reflects the transfer of ownership from the health sector to the education sector and a change, not only in terminology, but also in how health promotion is operationalised within schools. Health and well-being is now the responsibility of all staff within a school and has been afforded greater recognition and status in the curriculum. Furthermore, Government Education Inspectors have a formal requirement to review and report on the health promotion work of the school. This new phase is still in its infancy and it remains to be seen what impact Curriculum for Excellence will have on health and well-being in the longer term. Local authorities, schools and teachers are at different stages of understanding, acceptance, adoption and implementation. However, it demonstrates that in Scotland health promoting schools are becoming established in the mainstream of the education system (Young, 2005).

Reflections and lessons learned

The journey towards HPS implementation in Scotland highlights a number of factors as being crucial in facilitating this process. First, there is a need for political will and a supportive policy framework. Second, another important strategy evident within the Scottish context was the giving of power and autonomy to local authorities. Third, at a national level, clear aims and targets were set and resources provided while avoiding a top-down imposition of ideas and values that were not inherent to the local level. This has previously been described as 'contextual guidance' – a combination of internal self-organisation of systems at local level and external framing of options at national level (Willke, 2007). Fourth, partnership working was also an essential process in achieving successful HPS implementation. Partnerships can provide more efficient use of resources, facilitate exchange of knowledge and skills, and increase the capacity to take action. Finally, closely linked to the importance of partnership is the issue of ownership. Scotland succeeded in embedding HPS into the education system at national level and thus establishing ownership within the education sector and at school level. In conclusion, from the first HPS conference in Scotland in 1986 to the embedding of health and well-being within the new Curriculum for Excellence represents a period of almost 25 years demonstrating that implementation is 'a process, not an event' (Fixsen, Naoom, Blasé, Friedman & Wallace, 2005: 15). It is important to recognise the complexity of change at national and local level and the need to allow time for the political system and school systems to evolve and adapt to a new way of being and doing.

References

Fixsen, D. L., Naoom, S. F., Blasé, K. A., Friedman, R. M. & Wallace, F. (2005). *Implementation Research: A Synthesis of the Literature.* Tampa, FL: University of South Florida.

Grek, S. (2011). Interviewing the education policy elite in Scotland; a changing picture? *European Educational Research Journal, 10*(2), 233–241.

Gugglberger, L. (2011). *Phases of School Health Implementation in Scotland.* Vienna: LBIHPR.

Inchley, J. & Currie, C. (2003). *Promoting Healthy Eating in Schools using a Health Promoting School Approach.* Edinburgh: Child and Adolescent Health Research Unit, University of Edinburgh.

Inchley, J., Muldoon, J. & Currie, C. (2007). Becoming a health promoting school: evaluating the process of effective implementation in Scotland. *Health Promotion International, 22*(1), 65–71.

Koelen, M. A., Vaandrager, L. & Colomer, C. (2001). Health promotion research: dilemmas and challenges. *Journal of Epidemiology and Community Health, 55,* 257–262.

Learning and Teaching Scotland. (1999). *Health Education 5–14 National Guidelines.* Dundee: Learning and Teaching Scotland.

NSW Health Department (2001). *A Framework for Building Capacity to Improve Health.* Sydney: NSW Health Department.

Paulus, P. (2005). From the health promoting school to the good and healthy school: new developments in Germany. In S. Clift & B. B. Jensen (Eds), *The Health Promoting School: International Advances in Theory, Evaluation and Practice* (pp. 55–74). Copenhagen: Danish University Press.

Paulus, P. (2009). *Anschub.de – ein Programm zur Förderung der guten gesunden Schule [Anschub.de – A Programme to Promote the Good Healthy School].* Münster: Waxmann.

Paulus, P. & Gediga, G. (2010). Anschub.de. Bericht über erste Ergebnisse der Evaluation eines Programms zur Förderung der guten gesunden Schule [Anschub.de. Report of the initial evaluation results of a programme that promotes the good healthy school]. In P. Paulus (Ed.), *Bildungsförderung durch Gesundheit. Bestandsaufnahme und Perspektiven für eine gute gesunde Schule [Education Promotion through Health, Analysis and Perspectives of the Good Healthy School]* (pp. 309–325). Weinheim: Juventa.

Paulus, P. & Witteriede, H. (2008). *Schule – Gesundheit – Bildung. Bilanz und Perspektiven [School – Health – Education].* Dortmund: Bundesanstalt für Arbeitsschutz und Arbeitsmedizin.

Scottish Executive (2003). *Improving Health in Scotland: The Challenge.* Edinburgh: The Stationery Office.

Scottish Executive (2004). *A Curriculum for Excellence.* Edinburgh: Scottish Executive.

SHPSU (2004). *Being Well Doing Well: A Framework for Health Promoting Schools in Scotland.* Dundee: Scottish Health Promoting Schools Unit.

Scottish Office (1999). *Towards a Healthier Scotland – A White Paper on Health.* Edinburgh: The Stationery Office.

Stern, C., Ebel, C., Vaccaro, E. & Vorndran, O. (2006). *Bessere Qualität in allen Schulen. Praxisleitfaden zur Einführung des Selbstevaluationsinstruments SEIS in Schulen. [Better Quality in Schools. Best Practice Guide to Introduce the Self Evaluation Instrument SEIS in Schools].* Gütersloh: Verlag Bertelsmann Stiftung.

Suhrcke, M. & de Paz Nieves, C. (2011). *The Impact of Health and Health Behaviours on Educational Outcomes in High-income Countries: A Review of the Evidence.* Copenhagen: WHO.

Willke, H. (2007). *Smart Governance: Governing the Global Knowledge Society.* New York: Campus-Verlag, Frankfurt am Main.

Young, I. (2005). Health promotion in schools – a historical perspective. *Promotion & Education, 12*(3–4), 112–117.

Young, I. & Currie, C. (2009). The HBSC study in Scotland: can the study influence policy and practice in schools? *International Journal of Public Health, 54,* S271–277.

Young, I. & Lee, A. (2009). Scotland: sustaining the development of health-promoting schools: the experience of Scotland in the European context. *Case Studies in School Health Promotion,* Part 2, pp. 225–238.

Young, I. & Williams, T. (1989). *The Healthy School.* Scottish Health Education Group/ WHO Regional Office for Europe.

PART III

Conclusions

The chapter in this part highlights how socio-ecological models can contribute to explaining and understanding the impact of national and school level activities. In this chapter the editors summarise and identify how the concrete case studies support the hypothesised theoretical assumptions of implementation and system theories. Furthermore, needs for future developments at practice and research level are identified.

10

CROSS FERTILISATION OF NATIONAL EXPERIENCES AND NEED FOR FUTURE DEVELOPMENTS

Oddrun Samdal and Louise Rowling

Introduction

Health promoting schools is about creating a supportive environment for both development and learning. It includes, but is not limited to, the traditional health education approach covered in subjects addressing the cross-curricular topic of health (e.g. physical education, home economics, biology, social science and religion) (Samdal, 2008). While the health education approach frequently builds on pre-packaged programmes with clear objectives and activities, and linear step-by-step procedures (Deschesnes, Martin & Hill, 2003; Lister-Sharp *et al.*, 1999; Stewart-Brown, 2006); the health promoting school builds on the notion that schools should develop their change processes based on their individual needs and capacity, involving all relevant stakeholders. Therefore, when integrating the health promoting school approach into the school policy, an important criterion will be to ensure a systematic setting approach is taken by the whole school as outlined in Chapters 2 and 3.

To date, implementation of actions to create health promoting schools has been left to the practitioners, who may have varying practice based knowledge. This may influence implementation delivery and thereby result in great disparity in outcomes. Further, it may compromise the efficacy outcomes the organisational change processes aim to achieve through whole school change for health and learning. Dooris and Barry in Chapter 2 argued that the development of research and evaluation to inform effective implementation practice in settings has not kept pace with action. Of particular importance they highlighted the attention to contextual factors, and the critical role of implementation information in judging outcomes. Additionally, Dooris and Barry emphasised the need to identify strategies that will capture the synergistic interaction and impact of multiple interdependent interventions and systems that operate at different levels and spheres within the context of specific settings. Attention has to be given to the qualities of health promotion within the context, being empowering, collaborative, participatory, and conducted in partnership.

Health promoting schools is also about achieving educational change, which requires understanding of the educational settings, how they innovate and change and what influences this. For example, Clarke and Barry (2011) found that a contextual factor, lack of cohesion in the school community, impacted on the implementation. Health promoting school principles and actions therefore need to be integrated with actions relating to the core business of the school setting (Deschesnes, Couturier, Laberge & Campeau, 2010; Mohammadi, Rowling & Nutbeam, 2010; Rowling & Jeffreys, 2006). Building on Chen (1998) and Greenberg, Domitrovich, Graczyk & Zins (2006), Dooris and Barry in Chapter 2 highlighted four factors crucial to the success of an implementation process; the characteristic of the implementer (e.g. knowledge, skills and motivation), organisational context (e.g. structure, ethos, history, resources), intervention delivery (e.g. quality and availability of training, materials etc.) and the community context (environment, local policies, agencies and collaborations etc.).

In Chapter 3 Wolfgang Dür explained in more detail the complexity in the interaction between the organisation and the individuals in achieving behaviour change, which is a core focus of implementation of health promotion. Dür employed systems theory to help understand and exploit the organisational system of schools to simultaneously achieve health promotion and educational objectives. Aiming at modelling the relationship between the organisation and the individual, Dür presented von Foerster's (1984) four-factor model: the organisation, the individual, their social and material environments and the interaction between staff members (teachers) and users (students). The interaction factor in this model is new compared with most previous models described and highlights the importance of communication between the individuals in the organisation. Communication based on mutual respect and possibilities of being heard and listened to, is likely to be more effective in stimulating the wanted behaviour change as opposed to top-down instructions being given. In Dür's chapter the generic model is further translated into specific use for implementing health promoting schools. Again the individuals' perceptions of and reactions to the implementation process, and the importance of always keeping a close dialogue with and between the participants of the change process, is highlighted. The need for sufficient time for planning and developing readiness among the participants is underlined. Similarly the organisational structure and support is addressed and how this can best be adapted to support development of readiness, motivation and empowerment among the participants in the implementation process.

In Chapter 4 the results of a meta-analysis aimed at identifying globally applicable and specific implementation components for achieving health promoting school objectives found similar organisational and individual level components. Eight components were identified:

1. preparing and planning for school development;
2. policy and institutional anchoring;
3. professional development and learning;
4. leadership and management practices;
5. relational and organisational support context;
6. student participation;
7. partnership and networking;
8. sustainability.

Principles from organisational change theory were employed to describe the theory-driven mechanisms for each component, i.e. the rationale *why* each component is needed. In Chapter 5 a theoretical and empirical base for *what* types of actions are needed from practitioners to implement the identified eight components was elaborated.

Although presented separately, the components and their operationalisation identified in Chapters 4 and 5 are interdependent and may be seen to operate in parallel. The unique use of principles from organisational and individual behaviour change theories to explain the mechanisms of each component aims at demonstrating how the interplay between individuals and organisation is core to the success of the implementation, thereby supporting the key messages in Chapters 2 and 3, and Nutbeam and Harris' (2004) claim that there is no single theory or model that can adequately guide the development and implementation of a health promoting programme or policy. A theoretical rationale for each component provides a good basis for implementation aimed at identifying which processes are needed, and why. The identified components are relevant for a variety of health promoting school initiatives, i.e. independent of the health topic and how it is introduced. The components are thus applicable both when the initiative is taken at school level to implement a school developed, topic focused initiative and for a health promoting school policy implementation requested regionally or as part of a national programme. In any intervention approach emphasis needs to be given to stimulating the interplay between individual and organisational capacities represented by the eight components to achieve successful implementation of the health promoting change process (Deschesnes, Couturier *et al.*, 2010).

As demonstrated in Chapter 4, the eight components can be organised into three categories:

1. school leadership;
2. establishing readiness for change;
3. organisational context.

Establishing readiness for change addresses the building of individual motivation and preparedness for participation in the implementation process. Staff are key players in both initiation and implementation of concrete activities in school. Their commitment, values and attitudes are crucial to the effort and thereby the degree of implementation. The importance of alignment processes to develop teachers' commitment and investment in the programme is also highlighted in implementation research (Donaldson, 2001). Through the initiation phase it is therefore important to develop motivation and personal interest among the participants. A vital element in this process may be to develop a common understanding and language for the project, its ideas and priorities. This participation may vary depending on staff members' designated roles in the school. Hence, all members of the school community should participate in defining and developing the project's framework and actions. Consensus around these issues is important in order to create and maintain motivation and interest for the project. In line with the system theory presented in Chapter 3, the participants' motivation will also depend upon a cost-benefit analysis of how useful they evaluate the project to be compared to what they have to contribute.

The students are frequently considered the main target group for implementation of health promoting schools. Involving them in the implementation of actions is considered to be essential for the impact of the actions, and also specifically meets the basic aims of health promoting schools by facilitating empowering processes (Kickbusch, 2003). The European centred case study in Chapter 8 described how a systematic approach can be taken to ensure student participation. Similarly, the involvement of stakeholders through partnerships and networking is central to the success of the implementation and change process, as identified in Chapters 7 and 9.

School leadership and the *organisational context* capture the organisational structures supporting the implementation process. Leadership strategies in a health promoting school approach are important for both the establishment of readiness for change, and for the support structures in the organisational context. Readiness can be built by nurturing links between health promoting school objectives and the overall visions and goals of learning in school. This can, for example be stimulated through focused group discussions with staff and dialogues between individuals. The leadership also needs to apply management strategies to develop a supportive organisational context to facilitate the desired changes and behaviours. These include scheduling time for teachers and students to collaborate on planning and implementation of health promotion activities, and prioritising resources for teacher training and purchase of external competence or equipment needed to implement actions. The leadership component is in this way important for the facilitation of the organisational structures as well as stimulating the individual motivation and readiness for change, as also described in the Norwegian case study in Chapter 6.

The interdependency of the organisation and the individuals underscores the socio-ecological dynamic of the implementation components. The socio-ecological approach is frequently suggested as a core of successful implementation (Deschesnes, Trudeau & Kébé, 2010; Greenhalgh, Robert, Macfarlane, Bate &

Kyriakidou, 2004; Wandersman, 2009). Building on the socio-ecological perspective, change in organisational structures, contexts and processes are employed to achieve change in individual level behaviour and perceptions (Silins, Zarins & Mulford, 2002; Wang & Ahmed, 2003). Such an interaction further captures the overall aims of the health promoting school initiative, in that the aim is to build supportive contexts to promote individual level health behaviours and perceptions (St Leger, 2000). The interlinked implementation components can also be seen to capture the complexity of schools as systems (Keshavarz, Nutbeam, Rowling & Khavarpour, 2010; Shiell, Hawe & Gold, 2008), reinforcing perspectives on the importance of system theory in guiding the implementation of health promoting schools presented in Chapter 3. The complexity is seen in the balance between dependency and autonomy. For example, teachers are dependent on curriculum and school leadership regulations for some of their actions and aims. At the same time they are expected to organise learning activities for their students and initiate needed change processes without being told what to do and how to do it. Similarly students are dependent on their teachers in terms of what learning activities they are invited into and to what extent they are allowed to influence and plan their own learning activities. This is particularly important for implementing health promoting schools that are governed by educational rather than health objectives.

The chapters in Part I, and implementation research in general, have to a large extent emphasised the importance of support factors within the organisation, such as competence, resources, and collaborative culture. Adding the school factor level Deschesnes and colleagues (Deschesnes *et al.*, 2003; Deschesnes, Trudeau *et al.*, 2010) have identified the importance of national and intersectoral support and collaboration. This finding is confirmed and elaborated in the case studies in chapter 7 from Australia and England where the importance of national policy and curriculum documents for health promoting schools are demonstrated to be vital for the sustainability at national, state and school levels. Similarly the case studies from Germany and Scotland in Chapter 9 highlighted how national level policy support structures can be developed through a strong collaboration and partnership between the health and education sectors, such as initiating local level actions to develop good schools for both health and learning. Also, the case studies from Canada (Chapter 6) and Portugal (Chapter 8) demonstrated the relevance of national level systematic support and action to implement the components of leadership (Canada) and planning (Portugal). Not only systematic implementation at school level is vital to a successful implementation of health promoting schools, but regional and national actions represent crucial stimulation and support for the prioritising of health promotion at school level and the quality of its implementation, introducing a double loop implementation process.

Green and Kreuter (2005) have in their model for planning, implementing and evaluating health promotion demonstrated such a double loop process. Applied to school level health promotion, implementation requires a two step approach. First, teachers, need to be prepared and supported by the school leaders before they can proceed with implementation actions involving the students. That is, the school leadership needs to develop the teachers' motivation, skills and readiness for taking part in the health promotion implementation, and specifically with regard to student involvement, which will be their key responsibility, as outlined in Chapter 8. Similarly readiness of other relevant stakeholders such as parents and school health services needs to be developed. Organisational support factors that can facilitate the implementation process include professional development activities, curriculum time, and the establishment and involvement of collaborating networks and partners. Leadership initiated reinforcement factors are also needed. Reinforcement can be implemented through a continuing focus on alignment by inviting teachers and other stakeholders to provide inputs and assist in decision making around the prioritising of health promotion activities, and through the monitoring of teachers' activities to ensure that agreed priority to the implementation process is given. Viig and Wold (2005) have demonstrated how this double loop process at school level was relevant for the implementation of health promotion in Norwegian schools.

Based on the observation of the importance of national and regional support in the case studies and in some of the chapters in Part I, it seems reasonable to apply the double loop approach also to demonstrate the interaction between the national/regional and the school level. Figure 10.1 diagrammatically represents the important experience expressed in almost all the case studies that school level quality implementation was highly dependent on national and regional level policies and stimulation.

The case study from Portugal is a good example of how the relationship between national and school level action worked. Nationally an initiative was taken by the government to establish a committee to facilitate implementation of health promotion in Portuguese schools, represented in the far left hand box of Figure 10.1. The committee took leadership and initiated actions to develop personal readiness among school leaders, teachers and other stakeholders through visits to schools and regional school boards. In these visits training for why the initiative was important and how it could be planned and implemented, was provided. Through this process school leaders and teachers felt motivated and skilled to initiate action at school level. The committee also initiated organisational support by convincing the government that health promotion needed to be a compulsory part of the national curriculum. This decision further stimulated resources from the government to more systematic professional development courses for teachers as well as resources to all schools that provided a plan for health promotion activities. Through clear leadership and reinforcement the committee thus addressed both the individual and organisational level at school to stimulate the school leadership and teachers to take local action. Building on the double loop model presented at school level above (Green & Kreuter, 2005; Viig & Wold, 2005), the model in Figure 10.1 could have been developed into a

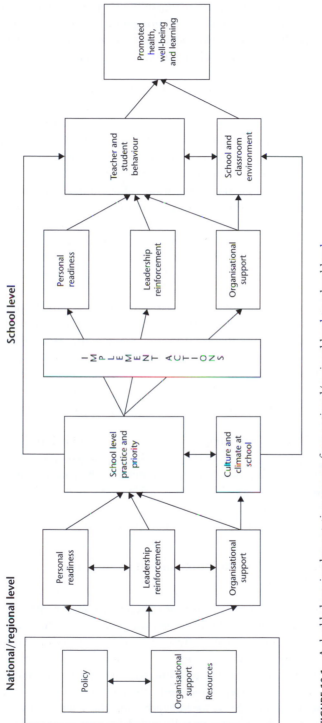

FIGURE 10.1 A double loop implementation process from national/regional level to school level

Source: Building on Green and Kreuter's (2005) Model for Planning, Implementing and Evaluating health promotion programmes and Viig and Wold (2005)

triple loop model to demonstrate more clearly how the Portuguese school and school leaders took the national implementation process further through stimulation of teachers' readiness and development organisational support structures and reinforcing actions to stimulate and facilitate teachers' implementation of student participation strategies and activities.

Similar to Portugal, the case study from Canada demonstrated the importance of systematic leadership at regional level for school level activities. In this case study the education and health sectors took important leadership roles that guided and initiated action at local schools. Also in the Scottish case study the importance of a national and regional support structure through a partnership for health promotion between the health sector and the education sector was described, culminating in a national education policy for health promotion. The curriculum is implemented through national and regional support systems. It is also part of the national monitoring of curriculum achievements, and thereby operates as an important national reinforcement factor for school level practice. A similar process of national support for school level action was presented in the English case study. Finally, the Australian and German case studies demonstrated how a national partnership organisation both influenced the national policy development and also represented an important organisational support structure for local schools in their efforts to implement health promotion in a manner that would help them build on and develop the principles of good educational standards. As individuals, as well as organisations, could be members, this was also likely to directly stimulate their readiness and motivation. The national member organisations further represent a key arena for reinforcing health promotion action at local level through sharing of experiences and ideas in the network.

Given the clear and positive impact of national and regional support it seems reasonable to encourage not only schools to use the identified components for implementation of health promoting schools, but also the national and regional support structures. In this way it will be possible to stimulate and continuously improve quality of action as the schools have a sparring partner to discuss activities with and receive continued support for their work.

How to achieve quality implementation of health promoting schools?

The identification of the evidence base for the eight components constituting the implementation system for health promoting schools signifies that it is not just the existence of the components to which attention needs to be paid, but also their functioning as a key outcome to be achieved (Rowling & Samdal, 2011), as addressed in Chapter 5. Recording the mechanisms of functioning of the implementation components and their elements in Chapters 4 and 5 is intended to provide a new focus for strengthening the science base for health promoting schools, as has been repeatedly called for over the past decade. The identification of implementation mechanisms through providing the theoretical and empirical rationale will serve three functions:

1. provide a complete theoretical framework for the implementation process;
2. stimulate quality practice;
3. provide basis for evaluation (see Figure 5.1 in Chapter 5).

The provision of a theoretical framework for implementation will help practitioners understand how the different components are interrelated and support each other. The interplay of individual and organisational components is particularly important to appreciate, as highlighted both by Dooris and Barry in Chapter 2 and Dür in Chapter 3. By understanding the interactions, the practitioners are likely to address the majority of the implementation components and not only the ones they themselves find most important or prefer working with. Further, knowing why a component is important or why a specific action is recommended to achieve the objectives of a component, will help practitioners to achieve quality practice with a sufficient standard of fidelity. Dür in Chapter 3 highlighted the importance of flexibility and room for adaptation in the implementation processes. Flexibility is expected to increase motivation for participation given that there is opportunity to use individual school audits of what is needed and fits their local context. But the need for flexibility cannot compromise what research shows are efficient and important means of change. Thus by knowing what the mechanisms of the suggested actions are, the practitioners become familiar with what they need to achieve. In this way they can more easily evaluate if their wanted adaptation will initiate the same mechanism or reach the desired objective. Finally, the identified operational mechanisms of each component will provide an important basis for evaluation of effectiveness and efficiency of the implementation process. In such an evaluation approach it is important to study the performance of the implementation process, i.e. the actions that have taken place, and to what extent that can explain achievement or lack of change.

Need for future developments

The complexity and dynamic nature of schools and the implementation of health promotion, which does not have the strict structure of a pre-packaged programme, has resulted in numerous debates and challenges about the form and focus of research and evaluation. These need to be attended to as a key element in improving implementation. A challenge for the future is therefore how to construct and conduct research and evaluation on all aspects of the implementation system, i.e. the separate implementation components and their interaction. This is a complex endeavour given the diversity of health promotion issues and differing individual and organisational facets where change can occur (Dooris and Barry, Chapter 2). Stewart-Brown (2006) concluded that few studies were identified that had used all the principles of health promoting schools. Similarly, the meta-analysis conducted to identify the implementation components that form the basis of this book (Chapter 4) did not identify any research/evaluation studies that included all the components of implementation.

To date mechanisms for researching and evaluating the diversity and complexity of the implementation system have not been found. There are two fields that researchers have identified as needing attention, the readiness not only of the individuals, but also of the system for change, that is, addressing and accommodating barriers and school conditions (Deschesnes, Nathalie & Couturer, in press; Inchley, Muldoon & Currie, 2007); and the documentation of the actions, processes and outcomes of implementation in the school and classroom. Dür in Chapter 3 concluded that there is a need to look at the relationships and exchange processes, between the organisation, the intervention and the individuals, but also between the individuals in the organisation. The implications are, that what is needed is to monitor and assess the interactional processes, the organisational conditions, and the outcomes at both individual and organisational level.

Dooris and Barry in Chapter 2 argued for different ways of conceptualising evaluation. They proposed two promising approaches, theory-driven research (Birckmayer & Weiss, 2000) and realist evaluation (Pawson, Greenhalgh, Harvey & Walshe, 2004), as ways to unpack the complexity of how programmes work or fail in particular settings. Another way of developing understanding of how programmes operate is through using Program Logic (Duignan, 2004). This allows for the sequence of actions – project inputs, process evaluation impact and outcome evaluations – to be tracked prospectively. That is, intended outcomes are identified in the planning stage, and their 'logic' links documented as the programme action provides implementation data. Analytical frameworks are needed to link the process with the impact and outcomes. Careful process monitoring provides for serendipitous events to be captured.

One of the themes running through this book is the need to conceptualise, implement and evaluate health promoting school practices in a different way to 'single' health topic interventions. In the past, single issue interventions have often ignored the context. This lack of attention to context can be partly explained by a clash of epistemology in health promoting schools research and evaluation. In education, the goal of 'evaluation' has usually been to provide information to enable an overall judgement of a programme (summative), in order that the programme can be improved and delivered (formative), and to identify any unintended consequences. Health science has emphasised the use of the randomised control trial (RCT) research design, with its linear cause and effect approach in determining the evaluation of effectiveness. However, this linear trajectory does not match health promotion practice with its more process, multi-component and multilevel approach. The resulting complexity involves identifying the linking elements, monitoring individual–organisation–intervention interaction and accommodating the dynamic nature of schools. Research designs are required to accommodate this complexity of factors that influence change in individuals and change in the school organisation, and the interplay of theory and practice, as well as research and practice.

While there is considerable development in the implementation science field, this is still almost exclusively focusing on the scaling up of pre-packaged programmes that have been trialled under health science research conditions. It is imperative that research be carried out to monitor implementation actions in naturalistic conditions. In doing this, attention needs to be paid to two forms of evidence, evidence-based practice and practice-based evidence. In schools, the latter involves pedagogical expertise that includes identifying and monitoring intellectual quality, relevance, supportive class environment and recognition of difference (Gore, Griffiths & Ladwig, 2004).

The areas of research and evaluation in need of development identified by Greenhalgh and colleagues (2005) are also relevant for further development of the science base for implementation of health promoting schools: namely theory driven research, a focus on process rather than 'package', greater emphasis on ecological analyses, a common language, measures and tools, collaboration and coordination, multidisciplinarity and multimethod research, meticulous details, and participation between practitioners and researchers. In the dynamic environments of schools there are a number of issues that can compromise the research and evaluation process. If researchers view schools as ideal 'contained' settings for data gathering under 'controlled' conditions without reciprocity in feeding back the data, i.e. 'raiding the schools for data', then long term data fatigue can occur in schools resulting in limited commitment to following research protocols. Participatory action research with schools as partners is respectful of the school's role in research, and their interest and need for the data to improve their practice (Hazell, Vincent, Waring & Lewin, 2002). The joint focus of simultaneously addressing research and practice needs for development is also highlighted by Nutbeam (1996) and Nutbeam and Bauman (2006). In addition they note the importance of involving policy interests and needs as part of the evaluation design to ensure priority is given to implementation of research findings.

Evaluations that capture the complexity of the school system and its importance for the implementation of health promoting schools will contribute not only to a better research base for the already identified, and possibly new components, for successful implementation. Such evaluations will also take evaluation science forward in that it identifies good ways of observing and studying the impact of the interplay and interaction between the individual and the organisation on implementation outcomes.

The development in the future of greater understanding of the complexities of health promotion practice and of school settings and their interaction, by both health and education sectors, holds promise for enhancing implementation theory, practice and research.

References

Birckmayer, J. & Weiss, C. (2000). Theory-based evaluation in practice. What do we learn? *Evaluation Review, 24,* 407–431.

Chen, H. (1998). Theory-drive evaluations. *Advances in Educational Productivity,* 7, 15–34.

Clarke, A. M. & Barry, M. M. (2011). *An Evaluation of the Zippy's Friends Emotional Wellbeing Programmeme for Primary Schools in Ireland.* PhD Thesis, Discipline of Health Promotion, National University of Ireland Galway.

Deschesnes, M., Couturier, Y., Laberge, S. & Campeau, L. (2010). How divergent conceptions among health and education stakeholders influence the dissemination of healthy schools in Quebec. *Health Promotion International, 25*(4), 435–443.

Deschesnes, M., Martin, C. & Hill, A. J. (2003). Comprehensive approaches to school health promotion: how to achieve broader implementation? *Health Promotion International, 18*(4), 387–396.

Deschesnes, M., Nathalie, D. & Couturer, Y. (in press). Schools' absorptive capacity to innovate in health promotion. *Journal of Health Organization and Management.*

Deschesnes, M., Trudeau, F. & Kébé, M. (2010). Factors influencing the adoption of a Health Promoting School approach in the province of Quebec, Canada. *Health Education Research, 25*(3), 438–450.

Donaldson, G. A. (2001). *Cultivating Leadership in Schools: Connecting People, Purpose, and Practice.* New York: Teachers College Press.

Duignan, P. (2004). The Use of Formative Evaluation by Government Agencies. http://www.strategicevaluation.info/se/documents/121pdff.html (accessed 12 March 2012).

Gore, J. M., Griffiths, T. & Ladwig, J. G. (2004). Towards better teaching: productive pedagogy as a framework for teacher education. *Teach Teacher Education,* 20, 375–387.

Green, L. W. & Kreuter, M. W. (2005). *Health Program Planning: An Educational and Ecological Approach* (4th edn). New York, NY: McGraw-Hill.

Greenberg, M. T., Domitrovich, C. E., Graczyk, P. A. & Zins, J. E. (2006). *The Study of Implementation in School-Based Prevention Research: Implications for Theory, Research, and Practice.* Rockville, MD: Centre for Mental Health Services, Substance Abuse and Mental Health Services Administration.

Greenhalgh, T., Robert, G., Bate, P., Kyrakidou, O., Macfarlane, F. & Peacock, R. (2005). *Diffusion of Innovations in Health Service Organisations: A Systematic Literature Review.* Oxford: Blackwell Publishing.

Greenhalgh, T., Robert, G., Macfarlane, F., Bate, P. & Kyriakidou, O. (2004). Diffusion of Innovations in Service Organizations: Systematic Review and Recommendations. *Milbank Quarterly, 82*(4), 581–629.

Hazell, T., Vincent, K., Waring, T. & Lewin, T. (2002). The challenges of evaluating national mental health promotion programs in schools: A case study using the evaluation of MindMatters. *International Journal of Mental Health Promotion, 4*(4), 21–27.

Inchley, J., Muldoon, J. & Currie, C. (2007). Becoming a health promoting school: evaluating the process of effective implementation in Scotland. *Health Promotion International, 22*(1), 65–71.

Keshavarz, N., Nutbeam, D., Rowling, L. & Khavarpour, F. (2010). Schools as social complex adaptive systems: A new way to understand the challenges of introducing the health promoting schools concept. *Social Science & Medicine, 70*(10), 1467–1474.

Kickbusch, I. (2003). The contribution of the World Health Organization to a new public health and health promotion. *American Journal of Public Health, 93*(3), 383–388.

Lister-Sharp, D., Chapman, S., Stewart-Brown, S. & Sowden, A. (1999). Health promoting schools and health promotion in school: two systematic reviews. *Health Technology Assessment 3*(22), 1–207.

Mohammadi, N. K., Rowling, L. & Nutbeam. (2010). Acknowledging educational perspectives on health promoting schools. *Health Education, 110*(4), 240–251.

Nutbeam, D. (1996). Achieving 'best practice' in health promotion: improving the fit between research and practice. *Health Education Research, 11*(3), 317–326.

Nutbeam, D. & Bauman, A. (2006). *Evaluation in a Nutshell: A Practical Guide to the Evaluation of Health Promotion Programs.* Sydney: McGraw-Hill.

Nutbeam, D. & Harris, E. (2004). *Theory in a Nutshell: A Practical Guide to Health Promotion theories.* Sydney: McGraw-Hill.

Pawson, R., Greenhalgh, T., Harvey, G. & Walshe, K. (2004). *Realist Synthesis: An Introduction. RMP Methods Paper 2/2004.* Manchester: ESRC Research Methods Programme, University of Manchester.

Rowling, L. & Jeffreys, V. (2006). Capturing complexity: integrating health and education research to inform health-promoting schools policy and practice. *Health Education Research, 21*(5), 705–718.

Rowling, L. & Samdal, O. (2011). Filling the black box of implementation for health-promoting schools. *Health Education, 111*(5), 347–366.

Samdal, O. (2008). School health promotion. In H. Heggenhougen (Ed.), *The Encyclopedia of Public Health* (Vol. 5, pp. 653–661). Oxford: Elsevier Inc.

Shiell, A., Hawe, P. & Gold, L. (2008). Complex interventions or complex systems? Implications for health economic evaluation. *British Medical Journal, 336*(7656), 1281–1283.

Silins, H., Zarins, S. & Mulford, B. (2002). What characteristics and processes define a school as a learning organisation? Is this a useful concept to apply to schools? *International Education Journal, 3*(1), 24–32.

St Leger, L. (2000). Reducing the barriers to the expansion of health promoting schools by focussing on teachers. *Health Education, 100*(2), 81–87.

Stewart-Brown, S. (2006). What is the evidence on school health promotion in improving health or preventing disease and, specifically, what is the effectiveness of the health promoting schools approach? *Health Evidence Network Report.* Copenhagen: WHO Regional Office for Europe.

Viig, N. G. & Wold, B. (2005). Facilitating teachers' participation in school-based health promotion – a qualitative study. *Scandinavian Journal of Educational Research, 49*(1), 83–109.

von Foerster, H. (1984). *Observing Systems (The Systems Inquiry Series).* Seaside, CA: Intersystems Publications.

Wandersman, A. (2009). Four keys to success (theory, implementation, evaluation, and resource/system support): high hopes and challenges in participation. *American Journal of Community Psychology, 43*(1), 3–21.

Wang, C. L. & Ahmed, P. K. (2003). Organisational learning: a critical review. *The Learning Organization, 10*(1), 8–17.

INDEX

Numbers in **bold** indicate figures and tables.

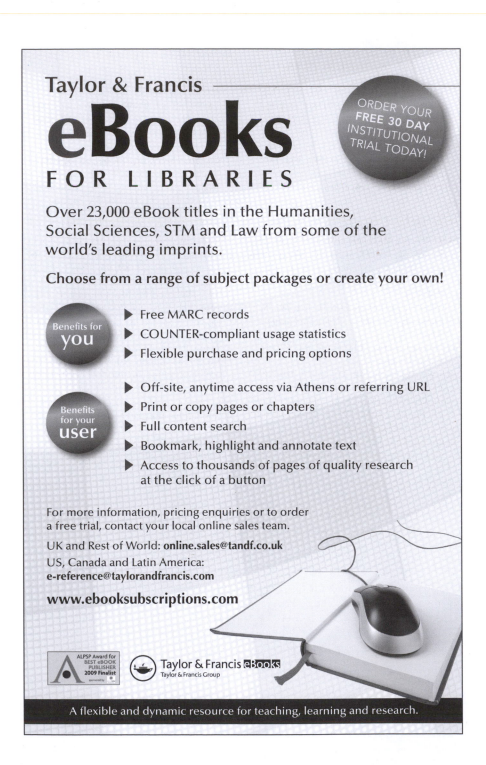